AROMATHERAPY FOR EVERYONE

By Jan Kuśmirek

CONTENTS

INTRODUCTION

Aromatherapy has become one of the world's most popular therapies for health, beauty and well-being. Its health giving benefits have become recognised in branches of orthodox medicine, nursing, midwifery and certainly in cosmetic science.

This book has been compiled together with the Fragrant Earth Academy to help the home user make the most of the essential oils used in Aromatherapy. It is not intended to be a comprehensive guide to the practice of Aromatherapy, which requires thorough professional training. Nor should this publication be regarded as a substitute for expert advice. For serious medical symptoms, you should always consult a qualified medical or complementary practitioner.

However, used correctly, essential oils can be used safely by your family and friends at home, at work or play as part of an aromatic and beneficial lifestyle. Aromatherapy is an invaluable aid to relaxation, stress relief, beauty care and to the improvement of health and well-being.

Within complementary medicine and cosmetology, Aromatherapy is an ever expanding field. There are a number of different training schools, each with its own particular emphasis. The information given here has been compiled from several different sources. It is intended for general interest and may not represent the actual views, policy or practice of the Fragrant Earth Academy.

WHAT IS AROMATHERAPY?

Aromatherapy is a natural treatment which uses the volatile molecules and concentrated herbal energies from plants and flowers which we call *'essential oils'*. They are used in association with massage, friction, inhalation, compresses and baths. An enjoyable experience in itself, it also improves and maintains well-being, health and beauty.

While many massage practitioners and relaxation experts use essential oils as an adjunct to their work, Aromatherapy is a holistic treatment in its own right. In the hands of qualified practitioners it can help to combat a wide range of physical and emotional problems. It has been shown to be successful not only in the treatment of stress-related conditions but also with muscular, circulatory, respiratory, digestive and skin problems and ailments. And, as this booklet describes, it can be used at home for relaxation, health and beauty care, and as safe support to other treatment in illness, for first aid, or simply to enhance the atmosphere at home or work.

Aromatherapy is a holistic form of healing which works with the body to promote health. Like other forms of holistic treatment, such as Homeopathy, Classical Aromatherapy does not work on the 'magic bullet' or 'pill popping' culture we have become familiar with in orthodox medicine, in which one chemical or drug is aimed at a specific disease. In fact, all essential oils have a wide range of applications.

If you visit a qualified Aromatherapist, he or she will first discover not only what your symptoms are, but what kind of person you are. You will be asked about your diet, lifestyle, and any stresses and strains in your life. Only then will the practitioner decided which oil or combination of oils will suit you best, and the choice may change from visit to visit as your well-being improves. Massage with the oils forms a major part of the treatment, but the Aromatherapist may also act as a counsellor, and advise on nutrition, exercise and other aspects of your health.

Now you can make life simple by using this easy to understand home care guide to essential oils. Discover the benefits of health giving natural fragrances – and yes its true – even smell alone can work wonders!

AROMAS, HERBS AND OILS THROUGH HISTORY

The use of aromatic materials for healing is as old as time. The medicinal properties of scented plants, flowers and woods were known to all the great ancient civilisations including Egypt, Babylon, China, India, Arabia, Greece and Rome.

The priest-physicians of ancient Egypt used Fragrances that we know today, such as Cedar Oil, in medicine, embalming, and in religious ceremonies. The ancient Greeks, who believed that perfumes were formulated by the Gods, used aromatic medicines and cosmetics, while the Romans used fragrant oils in massage. The word 'perfume' itself comes from the Latin 'par fumare', meaning 'through smoke' making reference to what we today would call incense.

In many Oriental cultures, the aromatic smoke burning of herbs had and still has religious and spiritual connotations, representing the prayers of worshippers and aiding the journey of the departing spirit at funerals. Scented herbs, oils and incense have also long been used in the Far East for both religious and medicinal purposes, while Native American Indians burned aromatic herbs to create smoke for their healing ceremonies.

Perfume and ointment makers have been involved for centuries in healing and promoting well-being. The Arabs, who specialised in using fragrant and aromatic substances, rediscovered the art of distilling and were among the first to use essential oils as we know them today.

In the West, the term 'essential oils' was coined by the 16th Century alchemists who were pursuing the 'quintessence', or secret of life; the ancient philosophers believed that there was a quintessential, or fifth element, which formed heavenly bodies and pervaded all things. Later the name was shortened to essential oils or essences. In 16th Century Germany, a physician called Jerome of Brunswick documented twenty-five essential oils, all still in use today.

In the late 17th Century, when herbs were used to combat pestilence and disease, herbalists like the famous Nicholas Culpeper used Essential oils including Peppermint in their medicines; in times of plague, people carried pomanders made with oranges and cloves to mask unpleasant smells and ward off infection but these were more than pretty smells. These pomanders contained disinfecting and germ killing oils!

Until the early part of this Century, all perfumes and many medicines relied on essential oils as their key ingredients; then cheaper synthetic and chemical flavourings and scents began to take over. Nonetheless, the finest perfume and soap manufacturers have continued to use essentials oils to give luxury products that quality which no imitation can match.

The revival of interest in essential oils began in the 1900's, with the French chemist René Gattefossé. He was working in the laboratory of his family's perfume business, when he burnt his hand badly. He plunged it into the nearest available liquid, which happened to be a bowl of neat Lavender oil. Not only did the burn heal astonishingly quickly, but there was no scarring. Impressed, Gattefossé began to research the healing properties of other essential oils, and published his book *'Aromatherapie'* in 1937.

In World War II the interest in Aromatherapy was pursued in France by Dr Jean Valnet, a medical doctor, who successfully used essential oils as internal treatment for wounded soldiers. At the same time, an Austrian biochemist, Marguerite Maury, was developing the use of essential oils with massage techniques especially for health and beauty.

During this period, the development of antibiotics and chemical antiseptics pushed the use of these powerful, natural oils into the background. Today, however, many people are disillusioned with synthetic, chemical ingredients in food, medicine, cosmetics and so on, and so we are witnessing a market turning towards healing methods that are natural, safe, and enjoyable.

Around the world, Aromatherapy has continued to be developed both by the orthodox medical profession as well as those in alternative and complementary practice. Numbers of nurses have trained in Aromatherapy and it is not uncommon to find Aromatherapy being offered in orthodox medical centres. Research studies in Europe, Australia and the United States among other countries show that essential oils used in Aromatherapy have definite therapeutic properties.

WHAT ARE ESSENTIAL OILS

Most of us are already familiar with essential oils in everyday life, probably without realising it. Each time we add a spice to a recipe, put mint sauce on roast lamb or crush a clove of garlic for a salad dressing, we are using essential oils. Many sweets are flavoured with essential oils or their derivatives; some liqueurs rely on them for characteristic flavours, including aniseed and caraway.

Essential oils, or 'essences', are the most potent form of a plant's aromatic and fragrant materials. They are obtained, usually by distillation, from the flowers, leaves, stems, bark or wood of aromatic plants and trees. For example, for Chamomile Oil the flower heads are used; for Lemon, the zest of the rind. Peppermint is made using the whole herb, and Sandalwood using the heartwood of the tree. Often huge amounts of raw material are needed to produce just a few drops of essential oil.

Essential oils are not oils in the everyday sense; they are not greasy or fatty. They are volatile, meaning they evaporate quickly. They are highly concentrated and extremely complex substances. Unlike vegetable oils like Olive Oil they leave little or no stain. Individual essential oils may contain many hundreds of chemical components, some in infinitesimal quantities, which all react together in a way impossible to reproduce synthetically. Essential oils are far more than pleasant-smelling perfume oils: they have specific actions, many of them medicinal. All of them are to some degree antiseptic, some (such as Tea Tree) quite powerfully so; some are also anti-viral and antibiotic; and so can help to combat infections.

Others are anti-inflammatory and can relieve both external burns and inflammatory conditions. Many are very useful in helping to stimulate the body's immune defence system and can be used not only for convalescence but also preventatively. Many are detoxifying and can help to clear congestion in the organs and lymphatic system.

Unlike drugs, some essential oils are particularly good at harmonising states of imbalance. Thus, when you read the descriptions of the individual oils, you will see that some have both a tonic and a sedative action, according to the state of the user. Also unlike drugs, many of the essential oils listed in this booklet have similar or overlapping properties. Thus you may find different properties for the same oils listed in different books.

How they work with body and mind

The newly expanding field of complementary and holistic medicine recognises the importance of the link between mind and body; that is, our emotional response to external stress has a direct effect on the body. How stresses affect us depends on our own constitution; some people may respond to stress with ulcers or digestive upsets, some with anxiety and insomnia, while others may develop high blood pressure. Holistic medicine takes into account the difference in symptoms and the individual stresses underlying them.

Essential oils appear to work on all levels, with both our physical body and also our psyche. In massage, their physical properties penetrate the skin and reach the bloodstream in tiny quantities to heal our muscles and organs. At the same time we are receiving their scents through the nose, whether through massage or other applications. It appears that they can activate a deep part of the brain, which stores memories, and that they also have an effect on the nervous system so that they can help to reduce anxiety, for instance - without the side effects of chemical tranquillisers.

THE IMPORTANCE OF QUALITY

To gain the best results only the best quality oils should be used, and they should be bought from a reputable source. Some oils are easier to obtain than others, so they vary in price; the rarest oils can be very expensive costing over a thousand British pound per kilogram. However, Aromatherapy is one area in which you really do get what you pay for; very cheap oils may be adulterated and offer little in the way of aroma or true benefit. Synthetic chemicals are used to mimic essential oils and are little more than chemical soups. Since quality oils are highly concentrated, a small bottle goes a long way.

True Rose is a good example of why essential oils are expensive. To make just 30 – 50 grams of Rose essential oil you would need 1 tonne of fresh flowers! No wonder chemists make cheap synthetic mimics. Where the plant is grown matters too. The best quality Lavender Oil, for example, is grown at a height above 3000 feet and due to this altitude contains a high level of the natural chemical Linalyl Acetate which produces the most relaxing oil. But much of the lavender used in poorer commercial essential oils is grown much closer to sea level and lacks this important constituent.

As essential oils are always diluted in a vegetable or 'carrier' oil when being used, some sensible and enlightened companies also sell ready blended or ready to use essential oils, which make for a more economic buy. This is also a safer way of buying essential oils as neat essential oils can cause problems of skin irritation. If buying this way, also make sure that the essential oil is the best quality for therapeutic use and not just a cheap fragrance oil.

A good true essential oil will come from a named botanic species and the aroma will be vigorous and lively, rather than simply strong. The extra sparkle and vitality of a top quality oil is always obvious in comparison with inferior oils.

Organic oils, because of the way they are grown, are sympathetic to the environment and sustainable too, making them a proper buy for those interested in the planets welfare. Organic means the produce may have come from naturally growing wild plants, or from wild crafted crops whose seeds have been sown in areas where the plant grows naturally. Other oils come from systems of biological or organic farming, a method which does not rely on synthetic chemicals for growth or pest control.

The aroma of the best oils varies naturally from year to year because of changes in climate, rainfall and soil conditions. So oils that smell exactly the same year after year are likely to have been altered in some artificial way to ensure a consistent aroma.

Carrier Oils: Essential oils are highly concentrated and as a rule should not be applied neat. For massage, Aromatherapists blend them with vegetable oils called 'carrier oils'. The best carrier oils are virgin cold-pressed oils which contain active vitamins and fatty acids; they do not have a powerful aroma of their own.
Those used by Aromatherapists include Sweet Almond, Walnut, Wheatgerm, Grapeseed, Jojoba, Apricot Kernel and Hazelnut. It is also possible, and

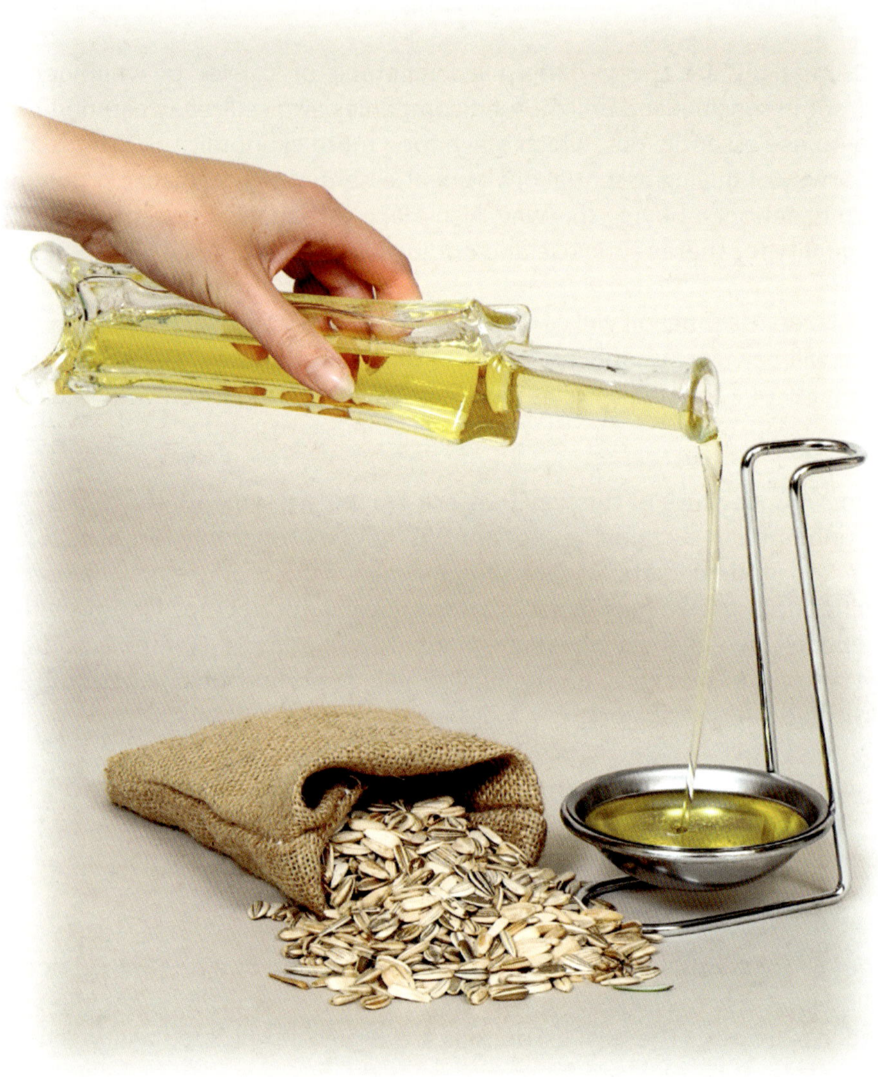

preferable to buy carrier oils specially pre-blended for the purpose.

Ready Blended essential oils can be bought ready mixed in a carrier oil, made up for specific purposes such as relaxation, baths, massaging aching muscles, and so on. Again, watch out for quality. A good quality pre-mixed, subtly fragrant oil can be very effective and provides a good introduction to the use of essential oils. The best are often called synergies rather than blends. The word 'synergy' itself implies that something not only works together but does more than expected!

STORING OILS

Always keep oils in the dark bottles in which they are supplied, in a cool, dry place away from any substances such a homeopathic medicines, which might be affected by the aroma. Keep the caps tightly closed to avoid evaporation. Unless you want your cheese to smell of an essential oil don't store them in the fridge!

When you make up your own blends, also store them in dark glass bottles (never plastic), and keep the caps tightly screwed on. They should keep for many months, stored in a cool place.

USING ESSENTIAL OILS AT HOME

Qualified Aromatherapists use essential oils to treat a surprising number of ailments. Since this booklet is intended for non-professional use, included are the main uses of a selection of oils which can be safely used at home, for yourself, family and friends.

While serious conditions should be treated by a qualified practitioner, many common ailments can be relieved safely and effectively at home with Aromatherapy. You may soon come to regard essential oils as a vital part of your home and first aid kit.

For self-help, essential oils are most commonly used to relieve aches and pains, for relaxation and stress reduction, and for skin and hair care, but they have much wider possibilities.

Many oils have proven antiseptic properties. They can be used as first aid and on-going treatment for cuts, burns, insect bites and bruises. Others are anti-inflammatory, anti-bacterial, antibiotic etc. Oils with anti-fungal properties can be used for such conditions as athlete's foot and other fungal infections.

Some can be used as an aid in the overall management of more serious conditions such as candida, arthritis and rheumatism.

In addition, since the oils work through the brain to act on the emotions, they are very useful not only for stress-relief, but in cases of anxiety, overwork, stage fright etc. Lists of oils recommended for specific physical and emotional symptoms are given on pages 21-37. While essential oils may help to alleviate symptoms, people suffering from serious conditions should always seek expert advice from a qualified Aromatherapist.

Caution should be exercised when using the oils to treat children, in pregnancy etc., and there are some people for whom Aromatherapy is not always suitable. Do take some time to read the Cautions section on pages 18/19; if in doubt, seek advice from a qualified practitioner.

Selecting oils
If you want to alleviate a specific problem, first look up your symptoms in the Index of Physical Symptoms on pages 21-30 and see which oils are recommended. Then, read the Index of Mental/Emotional Symptoms on pages 31-37. For example, if you are suffering from fatigue, are your symptoms accompanied by anxiety or depression, or caused by overwork? To complete the picture, read the descriptions of the recommended oils and see which come closest to your personal needs.

Since we are all individuals, some oils will be more appropriate to particular people than others. Enjoy experimenting with the oils; experience will help you to become more expert.

The sniff test: if you can, sniff essential oils before using them to make sure that they appeal to your sense of smell as fitting your other needs. Essential oils have a powerful aroma which can cause a strong reaction when you sniff them, especially if you sniff direct from an open bottle. The best way to test the scent of an oil is to put a single drop onto a handkerchief, and then gently inhale from that.

Blending oils

The concept of individuality is important in Aromatherapy, and it is rare for two people to react in exactly the same way. We can, however, generalise about the effects of particular essential oils which have specifications - for example, a particular group of plants may have anti-inflammatory properties, some are relaxing and sedative, some invigorating and so on. Blends of 2-3 oils can be made with these general characteristics to suit your personal needs.

Your chosen oils can be blended together and diluted in carrier oil, but do not exceed the total amounts recommended.

Oils bought ready blended in a carrier oil for general purposes, like baths, massage and room fragrance, will not require further dilution.

Using the oils

Once you have chosen a suitable oil or blend of oils, you can use them in the following ways:

Massage

Massage is a very effective way to relieve stress and tension. The ideal of course is to visit a professional Aromatherapist. However, for home care, massaging yourself or getting a partner to give you a gentle massage will still have benefits. Massage encourages circulation and eases minor aches and pains; it enables the essential oils to be absorbed and used by the skin and body. You do not have to have a full body massage to benefit; you can rub the blended oils locally into the area giving problems, whether it be muscular aches and pains, a stiff neck or a bronchitic chest. In self-massage, use gentle strokes towards the heart, to encourage the circulation. When massaging the abdomen, move your hands in clockwise circles, following the flow of the intestines; among other benefits, this helps to relieve constipation.

Making up Massage Oils

If you really want to make your own mix rather than use a ready to use product, choose a vegetable based carrier oil, preferably a blend of two or three oils with therapeutic properties of their own. Add 2 drops of your chosen essential oil/s to 5ml (1tsp) of carrier oil. Keep in a dark, stoppered glass bottle, and always recap tightly after use. The aroma will be taken up over a period of time, so the oil will smell more rounded after a week than just after it has been mixed.

Most oils are suitable for massage; for specific problems, see the indexes of symptoms. Bear in mind that some oils are relaxing and some stimulating.

Examples of recommended blends are:
- *For relaxation* - Geranium and Lavender
- *For aches and pains* - Juniper, Lemon, Rosemary
- *For cellulitis* - Juniper, Geranium and Rosemary

Baths

Bathing with essential oils is not just a pleasant way to relax; it can help to relieve many aches and pains and other physical conditions. Use a ready mixed blend, or use a maximum of 7-8 drops of pure oil to your bath, ideally at about 30°C, just before getting in. Stir the water well to disperse the oils. Do not use any other bath oil, salts or foam preparations at the same time. Close the windows and doors and relax in the water for ten minutes. You will benefit from the action of both the oil on your skin and in the water vapour.

Most oils are suitable for baths; however some of the stronger aromas, like Peppermint, may cause skin irritation. Check the recommended uses of the oils.

For children, use 2 drops of oil to a bath.

Footbaths

Add up to 5 drops of oil in a bowl of hand-hot water and soak the feet for ten minutes. Particularly suitable for tired and perspiring feet are Cypress, Juniper, Lemon and Tea Tree.

Sauna

Stir 3 or 4 drops of your chosen oil/s in water and then splash on the hot stones.

Inhalation/Facial Steaming

This way of using oils simultaneously gives your skin a cleansing treat while helping to clear congested lungs and sinuses, catarrh and sore throats.

On average use 2-3 drops to 1 pint of water. Float the oil on the surface of a bowl of steaming water, just off the boil. Drape a bath towel over your head and breathe in the steam for 2-3 minutes.

For nasal congestion, breathe through the nose; for a sore throat breath through the mouth. Do not persist if this causes a discomfort.

Exercise caution if you suffer from allergic conditions such as hayfever and asthma.

Compresses

Use *hot compresses* for long standing conditions like backache, arthritis and rheumatic pain.
Use *cold compresses* for recent injuries or acute conditions such as sprains, headaches, bruises and swelling.

For hot compresses, use water as hot as you can comfortably handle; for cold compresses, add ice to cold water. Add to the water up to 6 drops of essential oil, or 3 for small areas like the forehead. Fold a facecloth and place it on the surface of the water so that it takes up the essential oil. Wring out, and apply where needed (avoid getting
into the eyes).

Hair and Face Oil

Some oils are particularly good for the skin and hair (see List of Physical Symptoms). Use proportions of 1 drop of essential oil to 10ml (2tsp) carrier oil (preferably pre-blended for the purpose) for a pre-bath facial oil or as an after bath body lotion and moisturiser.

For hair conditioning, massage the blend into the scalp and leave for 15-30 minutes before shampooing.

Headlice can be successfully and pleasantly treated with a mixture of Eucalyptus or Tea Tree with Lavender and Rosemary, using 40 drops of essential oils to 100ml carrier oil. Apply to wet hair, massage well in and leave for an hour before shampooing and combing out with a fine toothed comb. Repeat as necessary.

Hair Rinse

After washing your hair, stir 1 drop of oil in the water in which you give your hair its final rinse, or make up a hair rinse as follows:

4 drops of essential oil to 1 litre water. Use a screw top bottle and shake well to disperse the oil each time you use it, as oil does not dissolve in water.

Suitable oils include Rosemary, Geranium and Rosewood for dark hair, or Chamomile and Lemon for fair hair.

Skin Lotion

Skin lotions/tonics can be made by adding 10 drops of essential oil to 50ml of spring water. Use a screw top bottle and shake well to disperse. Suitable oils are listed under 'Skin' in the Index of Physical Symptoms, page 29.

Mouthwash

Using a screw top bottle, mix 2 drops of oil with 285ml (½ pint) of spring water, shaking well to disperse the oil each time you use it.

For fresh breath, suitable oils include Peppermint and Lemon. For mouth infections and gum problems, use Tea Tree or Kunzea. Do not swallow the mouthwash.

Room Fragrance

Used as room fragrances, essential oils create a pleasant atmosphere; at the same time, specific oils will have an effect on your mood, creating a good ambience for meditation, work, relaxation, romance or sleep. Some will also help to fumigate the air in cases of infectious illnesses. There are several methods of using oils for room fragrance:

- Add a few drops of neat essential oil to a bowl of dried flowers or Pot Pourri.
- Add a few drops to drawer liners & padded clothes hangers.
- Put a couple of drops on a hot light bulb.
- Add a few drops to a ball of cotton wool and tuck it behind a warm radiator, or float 2 drops on a saucer of water near a warm radiator. Oil vaporisers are available today in a number of shops. Float a couple of drops of oil on water at the top of a bowl, and burn a night light underneath, to release the aroma into the air.

Most oils can be used for room fragrance. Some are particularly suitable for special purposes, including:

- *Meditation*: Cedarwood and Sandalwood.
- *Infection*: Peppermint (alone); Tea Tree (alone); Eucalyptus and Rosemary; Lavender and Lemon.
- *Romance*: Ylang Ylang, Geranium, Sandalwood.
- *Relaxation/Sleep*: Chamomile, Lavender, Sandalwood, Ylang Ylang.

On Handkerchiefs/Tissues
For colds, headaches, stuffiness, travel sickness etc. put a drop or two of your chosen essential oil on a handkerchief to sniff at intervals.

As an aid to sleep, put 1-2 drops on a handkerchief or tissue and place beside your bed or close to your pillow. You can put neat essential oil drops direct on the pillow, but do not let your skin come into contact with the neat oil.

Neat Application
As a general rule, do not apply neat oils to the skin as they can produce a skin reaction. However, for the relief of insect bites and stings, and to disinfect cuts, a drop or two of certain oils (e.g. Tea Tree, Lavender or Rosewood) can be used on the spot. Put 1-2 drops on cotton wool and dab gently.

SPECIAL USES

The hectic pace of life today makes particular demands on everyone. Women often have to combine work, home care and the demands of children. Modern life exacts an emotional toll on men too, while they also engage in types of work and sports that can place great demands on the body.

Aromatherapy can really help to redress the balance by soothing away the effects of a strenuous day, boosting self-confidence and inner strength.

For women, especially feminine oils are: Clary Sage, Geranium, Lavender, Marjoram, and Ylang Ylang.

For men, especially masculine oils are: Cypress, Frankincense, Lemon, Rosewood and oils with a dual aspect like Clary Sage and Geranium.

Essential oils that help to refresh and uplift are: Lavender, Lemon, Rosemary and Rosewood. Essential oils that help you feel warm and secure are: Chamomile, Clary Sage, Lavender, Orange and Ylang Ylang.

CAUTIONS

Essential oils are powerful, and should be used with care. When using the oils at home, follow the guidelines below:

- Aromatherapy can be very helpful during pregnancy and labour, but only under qualified guidance. If you are pregnant, you are strongly recommended to consult a qualified Aromatherapist.

- Some oils are stimulants, which may sometimes affect people suffering from epilepsy. Sufferers should seek medical advice before using essential oils.

- For babies and small children use in extra-dilute quantities.

- Keep bottles out of reach of children.

- Unless specifically indicated, do not apply neat oils directly on to the skin, as they can cause irritation.

- For the same reason, it is advisable to give yourself a patch test on a small area of skin when using your own blend. Note that certain drugs, stress and the menstrual cycle can also affect your sensitivity.

- Keep oils away from the eyes, and do not rub your eyes after handling them. If you should get any in your eyes, wash them out with plenty of fresh water; seek medical advice if necessary.

- Essential oils are flammable, so do not put them on or near a naked flame.

- Some are solvents and may damage certain plastics and polished wood surfaces.

- Never take the oils by mouth, unless under medical instructions.

- If you are taking homeopathic remedies, check with your practitioner before using essential oils, as it is believed that strong aromas can cancel the effects of homeopathic medicine.

- If you suffer from skin or other allergies, use the oils very carefully, and patch test before using widely. If you are unfortunate enough to have an allergic reaction to perfume, you are likely to be allergic to all essential oils. In this case, seek some other gentle form of therapy, such as Homeopathy or Bach Flower Remedies.

- If in any doubt at all, consult a qualified Aromatherapist.

(See the addresses of organisations on page 64.)

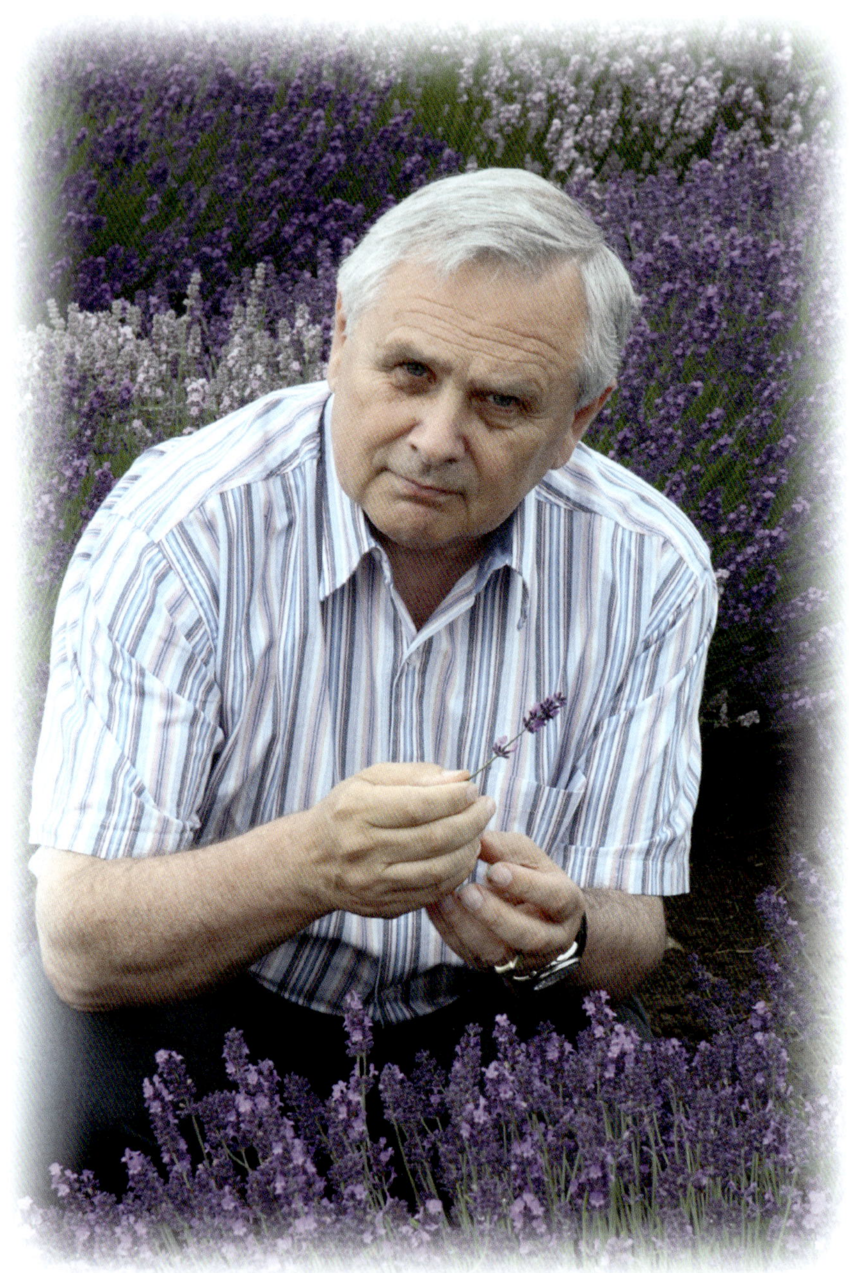

Jan Kuśmirek at The Somerset Lavender Farm, Faulkland, Somerset, UK.
Open to the public most of the year. www.somersetlavender.com

INDEX OF PHYSICAL SYMPTOMS

NB. These lists have been compiled from several sources.
Before using essential oils, read the Cautions on page 18/19.

If you are suffering from serious medical symptoms,
or if in any doubt, consult a qualified practitioner.

Most widely recommended.

SYMPTOM	RECOMMENDED OILS	HOW TO USE
Abscess, external **- Weeping**	Lavender, Tea Tree, Frankincense	Dab with 1-2 drops on cotton wool
Aches and Pains	*See Muscular Aches & Pains*	
Acne	*See Skin*	
Addictions	Clary Sage	Bath; massage; room fragrance/diffuser
Ageing, Problems of	Rosewood *See also Menopause*	Bath; massage; room fragrance/diffuser
Anaemia	Lemon	Bath; massage
Appetite, Loss of	Chamomile	Bath; massage
Arthritis **- Swollen Joints**	Chamomile, Cypress, Juniper, Lavender, Lemon, Marjoram, Rosemary, Ginger, Kunzea Juniper	Bath; compress; massage/rub affected area with massage oil
Asthma	Cedarwood, Clary Sage, Eucalyptus, Lavender, Lemon, Nerolina, Marjoram	Bath; massage/rub with massage oil. Avoid inhalations
Athlete's Foot	Lavender, Lemon, *Tea Tree	Foot bath; dab with 1-2 drops on cotton wool
Backache	*See Lumbar Pain, Muscular Aches and Pains*	
Baldness/Hair Loss	Clary Sage, Lavender, *Rosemary, Ylang Ylang	Scalp Oil
Bedwetting	Chamomile, Cypress, Lavender	Bath; massage
Bites	*See Insect Bites*	
Blisters	Lavender	Dab with 1-2 drops on cotton wool
Blood Pressure **- High/Low**	Clary Sage, *Lavender, Lemon, Marjoram, *Ylang Ylang, Rosemary	Bath; massage

SYMPTOM	RECOMMENDED OILS	HOW TO USE
Body Odour	Clary Sage, Cypress, Juniper, Lemon, Rosewood	Bath; massage, skin lotion
Boils	Chamomile, Juniper, Lavender, Lemon, Tea Tree	Bath; compress; dab with 1-2 drops on cotton wool
Breath, Bad	Kunzea, Lavender, Tea Tree	Mouthwash
Bronchitis	Cedarwood, Eucalyptus, Frankincense, Marjoram, Orange, Sandalwood, Tangerine, *Tea Tree, Ginger	Bath; inhalation; massage/rub chest with massage oil
Bruises	*Lavender, Tea Tree	Bath; compress; dab with 1-2 drops on cotton wool
Burns	*Lavender, Chamomile, *Tea Tree, Eucalyptus	Bath; compress; for small burns apply neat
Candida Albicans	Tea Tree	Bath; compress; massage
Catarrh	Cedarwood, Eucalyptus, Frankincense, Lavender, Lemon, Peppermint, Rosemary, Sandalwood, Tea Tree, Ginger	Bath; compress; inhalation
Cellulitis	Cypress, *Geranium, Juniper, Lavender, *Lemon, Rosemary, Red Grapefruit, Patchouli	Bath; massage/rub with massage oil
Chilblains - Itchy	Cypress, Juniper, Lavender, Lemon, Marjoram, Rosemary, Chamomile *See also Circulation, poor*	Bath; compress, footbath; dab with massage oil
Chilliness	Cypress, Frankincense, Marjoram, Rosemary	Bath; massage/rub with massage oil
Circulation, poor	Cypress, Juniper, Lemon, Marjoram, Orange, *Rosemary	Bath; massage/rub affected area with massage oil
Cold Sores	Eucalyptus, Tea Tree	Dab with 1-2 drops on cotton wool

SYMPTOM	RECOMMENDED OILS	HOW TO USE
Colds - **With sneezing**	*Eucalyptus, Lavender, Lemon, Marjoram, Orange, Tangerine, *Tea Tree, Rosemary	Bath; massage/rub throat and chest with massage oil; inhalation; room fragrance/diffuser
Colic	Chamomile, Juniper, Lavender, Sandalwood	Bath; massage/rub abdomen with massage oil
Colitis	Rosemary	Bath; massage/rub affected area with massage oil
Constipation	*Rosemary, Marjoram, Peppermint, Orange, Tangerine, Ylang Ylang, Ginger	Bath; massage/rub abdomen clockwise with massage oil
Convalescence	Clary Sage	Bath; massage; room fragrance/diffuser
Corns	Lavender, *Lemon, Marjoram, Peppermint	Dab with 1-2 drops on cotton wool
Coughs - **Bronchitic** - **Dry** - **Spasmodic**	Cedarwood, Eucalyptus, Frankincense, Ginger, Lavender, Lemon, Marjoram, Sandalwood Cypress Cypress, Lavender, Sandalwood Cypress, Nerolina	Bath; inhalation; massage/rub throat and chest with massage oil; room fragrance/diffuser
Cramp - **After exercise**	Clary Sage, Cypress, Juniper Rosemary, Marjoram	Bath; massage/rub with massage oil
Cuts	Eucalyptus, Lavender, *Tea Tree	Compress; dab with 1-2 drops on cotton wool
Cystitis	Chamomile, Cypress, *Tea Tree, Cedarwood, *Juniper, Eucalyptus, Frankincense, *Lavender, *Sandalwood	Hot compress; massage/rub abdomen with massage oil
Dandruff - **With oily scalp**	Cedarwood, Lavender, Rosemary, Tangerine Cypress	Hair oil; rinse

SYMPTOM	RECOMMENDED OILS	HOW TO USE
Dermatitis	*Chamomile, Geranium, Nerolina, Orange, Tangerine, *Tea Tree	Bath; compress; apply massage oil to affected area
Diarrhoea	Chamomile, Cypress, Eucalyptus, Geranium, Lavender, Peppermint, Rosemary, Sandalwood	Compress; massage
Earache	Chamomile, Lavender	Compress or cotton bud in ear with one drop of massage oil
Eczema - Weeping	*Chamomile, Geranium, *Lavender, Patchouli, Sandalwood Juniper, Lavender	Bath; apply massage oil to affected areas after patch test. *See Cautions, page 18/19*
Energy, Lack of	Orange *See also Exhaustion, Fatigue*	Bath; massage; room fragrance/diffuser
Exhaustion	Clary Sage, Frankincense, Lavender	Bath; massage; room fragrance/diffuser
Fatigue	Geranium, Marjoram, Peppermint, Rosemary	Bath; massage; room fragrance/diffuser
Feet, sweaty -Deodorants for	Cypress, Tea Tree Cypress, Juniper, Lemon	Bath; footbath
Feet, tired	Peppermint	Footbath
Flatulence	Ginger, Red Grapefruit, Marjoram, Peppermint, Tangerine	Massage abdomen
Fluid retention	Eucalyptus, Geranium, *Juniper, Lavender, Rosemary, Sandalwood, Patchouli	Bath; massage
Frigidity	Clary Sage, Rosewood, Sandalwood, Ylang Ylang	Bath; massage; room fragrance/diffuser
Fungal Infections	Geranium, *Tea Tree	Bath; compress; dab with 1-2 drops on cotton wool

SYMPTOM	RECOMMENDED OILS	HOW TO USE
Gastritis	Lavender, Peppermint, Tea Tree	Bath; massage/rub abdomen with massage oil
Gum Infections	Cypress, Kunzea, Tea Tree	Mouthwash
Haemorrhoids (Piles)	*Cypress, Frankincense, Juniper	Bath; general massage
Hair Care **- Dry** **- Oily/greasy**	Chamomile, Rosemary Geranium, Lavender, Sandalwood Clary Sage, Lemon *See also Baldness, Dandruff, Headlice*	Hair rinse; hair oil
Hangover	Juniper, Rosemary	Bath; inhalation; massage
Hayfever	Juniper	Drops on tissue; rub massage oil on sinuses
Headache **- Congestive** **- With Sinusitis** **- Tension**	Clary Sage, *Lavender, Rosemary, Marjoram, Peppermint Eucalyptus, Marjoram Eucalyptus Chamomile	Bath; compress; inhalation; massage or apply oil to head, neck and shoulders
Headlice	Geranium, Lavender, Tea Tree *NB: Avoid getting oil in the eyes*	Scalp oil
Hot Flushes	Chamomile, Lavender	Bath; massage; room fragrance/diffuser
Immune Deficiency (Recurrent infections)	Lavender, Lemon, Rosewood, Sandalwood, Tea Tree	Bath; massage; room fragrance/diffuser
Impotence	Clary Sage, Rosewood, Sandalwood, *Ylang Ylang	Bath; massage; room fragrance/diffuser
Indigestion	Chamomile, Juniper, Lemon, Peppermint, Orange, Sandalwood, Tangerine	Bath; massage/rub locally with massage oil
Infections	Nerolina, Tea Tree	Room fragrance/diffuser
Influenza	Cypress, Eucalyptus, Juniper, Kunzea, Lavender, Lemon, Nerolina, Peppermint, Tea Tree	Bath; inhalation; massage; room fragrance/diffuser

SYMPTOM	RECOMMENDED OILS	HOW TO USE
Insect Bites/Stings	Chamomile, Lavender, Lemon, Tea Tree	Apply 1 or 2 drops neat; bath; compress
Insomnia **- When physically tired**	Chamomile, *Lavender, Marjoram, Orange, Sandalwood, Tangerine, Ylang Ylang, Clary Sage *See also under Mental/Emotional symptoms for conditions causing the insomnia e.g. Anxiety, Depression etc.*	Bath; massage; room fragrance; 1 or 2 drops on a tissue beside the pillow
Irritable Bowel	Chamomile	Bath; massage abdomen
Joints; Painful **- Swollen** ***See also Arthritis, Rheumatism***	Lavender, Juniper, Rosemary Chamomile, Lavender	Bath; compress (cold for recent injury, hot for chronic pain); massage/rub affected area with massage oil
Laryngitis	Cypress, Lemon, Sandalwood	Bath; compress; inhalation; rub massage oil on throat and chest
Liver Problems	Chamomile, Geranium, Juniper, Rosemary, Tangerine	Bath; massage/rub affected area with massage oil
Lumbar Pain	Chamomile, Kunzea, Lavender, Rosemary	Bath; compress; massage/rub affected area with massage oil
Lymphatic Congestion	*Rosemary, Geranium, Lavender	Bath; massage/rub with massage oil
Menopause	Chamomile, Clary Sage, Cypress, Geranium, Lavender, Sandalwood	Bath; inhalation; massage
Menstrual Problems	*See PMT, Periods*	
Migraine	Chamomile, Clary Sage, *Lavender, *Marjoram, *Peppermint, *Rosemary	Bath; massage head and neck; inhalation; room fragrance/ diffuser
Mouth Infections	Geranium, Kunzea, *Tea Tree	Mouthwash
Mouth Ulcers **- External**	Lemon, *Tea Tree	Mouthwash; Dab with 1-2 drops on cotton wool

SYMPTOM	RECOMMENDED OILS	HOW TO USE
Muscle Spasm	Clary Sage	Rub with massage oil
Muscular Aches and Pains	Chamomile, Eucalyptus, Juniper, Kunzea, Lavender, Lemon, Marjoram, Peppermint, Ginger, Orange, Rosemary, Tangerine	Bath; compress; massage/rub affected area with massage oil
- After Sport	Chamomile, Marjoram	
Nausea	Ginger, Red Grapefruit, Lavender, Peppermint, Rosewood	Bath; inhalation
Nettle Rash	Chamomile, Tea Tree	Bath; compress; apply massage oil to affected area after patch test *See Cautions, page 18/19*
Neuralgia	Chamomile, Eucalyptus, Geranium, Lemon	Bath; compress; massage/rub affected area with massage Oil
Nosebleed	Cypress, Frankincense, Lavender, Lemon	Compress
Periods, Heavy	Cypress	Bath; compress; massage/rub abdomen with massage oil
- Irregular	Chamomile, Clary Sage, Geranium, Lavender	
- Painful	Chamomile, Clary Sage, Cypress, Juniper, Rosemary	
- Scanty	Juniper, Lavender	
Perspiration		Bath; massage; skin lotion
- Excessive	Clary Sage, Cypress	
Deodorants for,	*See Body Odour*	
PMT **(Pre-Menstrual Tension)**	Clary Sage, Chamomile, Geranium, Rosemary	Bath; compress; massage
- Painful Breasts	Geranium *See also Fluid Retention*	
Psoriasis	Geranium, Juniper, Lavender, Tea Tree	Bath; compress; apply massage oil to affected areas after patch test. *See Cautions, page 18/19*

SYMPTOM	RECOMMENDED OILS	HOW TO USE
Respiratory Problems	Cedarwood, Eucalyptus, Frankincense, Peppermint, Rosemary, Sandalwood	Bath; compress; inhalation; massage/rub chest and throat with massage oil; room fragrance/diffuser
Rheumatism	Chamomile, Cypress, Red Grapefruit, Juniper, Lemon, Lavender, Marjoram, Kunzea, Rosemary, Ginger	Bath; compress; massage/rub affected area with massage oil
Sciatica	Eucalyptus, Juniper, Kunzea *See also Muscular Aches and Pains, Rheumatism*	Bath; compress; massage/rub affected area with massage oil
Sexual Problems	Clary Sage, Rosewood, Sandalwood, *Ylang Ylang	Bath; massage; room fragrance/diffuser
Sinusitis	Eucalyptus, Lavender, Marjoram, Peppermint, Orange, Tea Tree	Bath; inhalation; compress; apply massage oil to sinus area
Skin Care and Problems		Bath; compress; massage; skin lotion
- **Acne**	Cedarwood, Chamomile, Geranium, Red Grapefruit, Juniper, Lavender, Tea Tree, Patchouli	
- **Ageing/Mature**	Clary Sage, Cypress, Frankincense, *Geranium, Lavender, Lemon, Orange, *Rosewood, *Sandalwood, Tangerine	
- **Allergies**	Chamomile	
- **Blackheads**	Peppermint	
- **Blotchy**	Geranium	
- **Broken Veins**	Cypress, Lemon, Chamomile	
- **Cracked**	Frankincense, Patchouli	
- **Dry**	Geranium, Lavender, Orange, *Sandalwood, Tangerine	
- **Greasy**	Lemon, Peppermint	
- **Infections**	Tea Tree	
- **Inflamed**	Chamomile, Clary Sage, Frankincense, Geranium, Lavender, Sandalwood, Tea Tree	

SYMPTOM	RECOMMENDED OILS	HOW TO USE
- Irritated/Itchy	Cedarwood, Chamomile, Lavender, Sandalwood	Bath; compress; massage; skin lotion
- Oily	Cedarwood, Cypress, Geranium, Juniper, Rosemary, Ylang Ylang	
- Sensitive	Geranium *See also Dermatitis, Eczema*	
Sprains	Chamomile, Lavender	Cold compress
Sunburn	Lavender	Bath; cold compress
Sweating, Excessive	Cypress *See also Body Odour*	Bath; massage
Throat		Bath; compress; rub massage oil on throat and upper chest
- Burning	Lavender	
- Dry	Lavender	
- Infections	Clary Sage, Geranium, *Tea Tree Sandalwood	
- Sore	Clary Sage, Lavender, Lemon, Sandalwood, Tea Tree	
Thrush	Tea Tree	Bath
Tinnitus	Lavender, Sandalwood	Compress
Toothache	Chamomile, Peppermint	Compress; mouthwash
Travel Sickness	Ginger, Lavender, Peppermint	Sniff a drop or two on a tissue
Urination		Bath; massage/rub abdomen with massage oil
- Frequent	Cypress	
- Painful	Juniper, Lavender *See also Cystitis*	
Varicose Veins	Cypress, Lemon, Patchouli	Bath; compress
Veruccas	Lemon, Tea Tree	Dab with neat oil
Warts	Lemon, Tea Tree	Dab with neat oil
Wounds	Lavender, Tea Tree	Bath; compress; can be applied neat

INDEX OF
MENTAL/EMOTIONAL SYMPTOMS

NB. This list has been compiled from several sources.
For mental and emotional states, the appropriate oils can
be used in baths, inhalation, massage and room fragrance.
A drop on a handkerchief or tissue can also be used.

MENTAL/EMOTIONAL SYMPTOMS	**RECOMMENDED OILS**
Absent-Mindedness	Cedarwood
Ageing, Feelings of	Tangerine
Anger	Chamomile, Peppermint, Ylang Ylang, Grapefruit
Anxiety	Cedarwood, Chamomile, Clary Sage, Frankincense, Geranium, Lavender, Marjoram, Rosewood, Sandalwood, Tangerine
- Sexual	Sandalwood, Ylang Ylang, Patchouli
Apathy	Lemon, Orange, Tangerine, Tea Tree
Bitterness	Lemon
Boredom	Orange
Burn-out	Frankincense
Change - Coping with - Difficulty in adjusting to - Difficulty in making	 Ylang Ylang, Nerolina Clary Sage, Nerolina Orange, Kunzea
Claustrophobia	Clary Sage, Frankincense
Compulsiveness	Clary Sage
Concentration, Lack of	Cedarwood, Eucalyptus, Rosemary, Kunzea
Confidence, Lack of	Ylang Ylang, Ginger
Confusion	Geranium, Lemon
Courage, Lack of *See also Fear*	Frankincense
Critical of Others	Rosewood
Cynicism	Sandalwood
Daydreaming	Cedarwood, Rosewood, Kunzea

MENTAL/EMOTIONAL SYMPTOMS	**RECOMMENDED OILS**
Depression	Chamomile, Clary Sage, Frankincense, Geranium, Lavender, Orange, Sandalwood, Tangerine, Ylang Ylang
Despondency	Juniper
Detail, Over-Preoccupation with	Tea Tree
Discipline, Lack of	Frankincense
Disorientation	Rosemary
Dreams, Recurrent	Clary Sage, Sandalwood
Empathy, Lack of	Rosewood
Emptiness, Emotional	Tangerine
Exhaustion, Mental	Frankincense
- From overwork	Clary Sage, Orange
Fatigue, Mental	Frankincense, Lavender, Peppermint, Rosemary, Rosewood
Fear	Chamomile, Frankincense
- Acute	Geranium, Nerolina
- Of coming events	Sandalwood
- Of confronting issues	Marjoram
- Of the dark	Lavender
- Of dying	Tangerine
- Of effort	Sandalwood
- Of failure	Lavender, Sandalwood, Ylang Ylang
- Of going mad	Ylang Ylang
- Of letting go	Cypress, Nerolina
- Of people	Geranium
- Of others' opinions	Cypress
- Rigid with	Geranium
- Of showing feelings	Marjoram, Ylang Ylang
- With inner trembling	Lavender, Nerolina
- Of unknown origin	Lavender
Frustration	Ylang Ylang

MENTAL/EMOTIONAL SYMPTOMS	RECOMMENDED OILS
Giving in to Others	Cypress
Grief - For lost past - Prolonged after loss	Marjoram Tangerine Frankincense
Grudgingness	Lemon
Grumpiness	Rosewood
Guilt Feelings	Juniper, Ylang Ylang
Hopelessness	Orange
Hostility	Clary Sage, Marjoram
Hyperactivity	Clary Sage, Lavender
Hypersensitivity	Peppermint
Hysteria	Chamomile, Lavender, Peppermint, Kunzea
Impatience	Chamomile, Lavender, Ylang Ylang
Impulsiveness	Chamomile
Indecision	Rosemary, Kunzea
Insecurity	Frankincense, Lavender, Sandalwood
Insomnia	Chamomile, Clary Sage, Lavender, Orange, Sandalwood, Tangerine, Ylang Ylang, Nerolina
Insatiability	Geranium, Rosewood
Irrationality	Lavender, Ylang Ylang
Irritability	Chamomile, Cypress, Lavender, Marjoram, Sandalwood, Ylang Ylang
Jealousy	Cypress, Ylang Ylang
Joy, Lack of	Orange, Tangerine

MENTAL/EMOTIONAL SYMPTOMS	RECOMMENDED OILS
Lethargy, Listlessness	Clary Sage, Cypress, Juniper, Lemon, Orange, Rosemary, Sandalwood
Loneliness	Marjoram
Memory, Poor	Rosemary
Moodiness, Mood Swings	Eucalyptus, Geranium, Lavender, Rosewood
Nerves: **- Exhausted** **- Living on**	Chamomile, Clary Sage, Juniper, Lavender Marjoram, Rosemary, Grapefruit, Kunzea Chamomile *See also Tension, Nervous*
Nightmares	Frankincense, Lavender
Nostalgia, Living in Past	Frankincense, Sandalwood, Tangerine
Obsession **-With past**	Clary Sage, Sandalwood Frankincense, Sandalwood
Obstinacy	Orange, Rosewood, Ylang Ylang
Overactive Mind	Chamomile, Lavender, Marjoram, Nerolina
Overburdened **- By responsibilities**	Rosewood Rosemary
Over-Emotional	Eucalyptus
Over-Talkativeness	Cypress
Overwork **- Mental strain from**	Lavender, Rosewood Clary Sage, Rosemary
Palpitations, Nervous	Lavender
Panic Attacks	Clary Sage, Frankincense, Lavender, Ylang Ylang, Nerolina
Paranoia	Frankincense, Lavender
Perseverance, Lack of	Frankincense
Procrastination	Sandalwood, Ginger

MENTAL/EMOTIONAL SYMPTOMS — RECOMMENDED OILS

MENTAL/EMOTIONAL SYMPTOMS	RECOMMENDED OILS
Resentment	Clary Sage, Lemon, Sandalwood, Ylang Ylang
Resignation	Orange
Restlessness	Chamomile, Lavender
Rigidity, Mental	Geranium, Rosewood
Sadness	Marjoram, Orange
Selfishness, Self-Centredness	Lemon, Orange, Sandalwood
Self-Criticism	Frankincense
Self-Esteem, Self-Worth, Lack of	Juniper, Rosemary, Sandalwood, Ylang Ylang
Sensitivity	Lemon, Sandalwood, Ylang Ylang
Shock	Tea Tree, Ylang Ylang, Kunzea
Shyness	Peppermint, Ylang Ylang
Stability, Need for	Frankincense
Stage Fright	Lavender
Strain, Mental	Chamomile, Clary Sage, Marjoram, Rosemary, Kunzea
Stress, General	Cedarwood, Chamomile, Clary Sage, Geranium, Juniper, Lavender, Marjoram, Tangerine, Grapefruit
Sulkiness	Clary Sage, Rosewood
Suspiciousness	Ylang Ylang
Tantrums in Children	Chamomile
Tension, Nervous	Cedarwood, Chamomile, Clary Sage, Cypress, Frankincense, Geranium, Juniper, Lavender, Rosewood, Sandalwood, Kunzea, Tangerine, Ylang Ylang, Grapefruit, Nerolina

Thoughts
- **Gloomy** — Orange
- **Irrational** — Marjoram
- **Negative** — Clary Sage, Lavender
- **Not in Present** — Cedarwood, Patchouli
- **Overactive** — Clary Sage, Lavender
- **Over-analytical** — Clary Sage
- **Racing** — Clary Sage
- **Restless** — Chamomile
- **Scattered** — Cedarwood
- **Unclear** — Eucalyptus, Lemon, Juniper, Peppermint, Rosemary

Touchiness — Lemon

Uncleanness, Feelings of — Tea Tree

Unforgivingness, Feelings of — Sandalwood

Unyielding to Circumstances — Rosewood

Weak-Willed — Cypress, Kunzea

Withdrawnness — Marjoram

Worry — Chamomile, Nerolina
- *About future* — Lavender, Sandalwood
- *About past* — Frankincense

TWENTY-FOUR OILS AND THEIR USES

Before using any oil,
read the Cautions on page 18/19.

CEDARWOOD *Cedrus Atlantica*

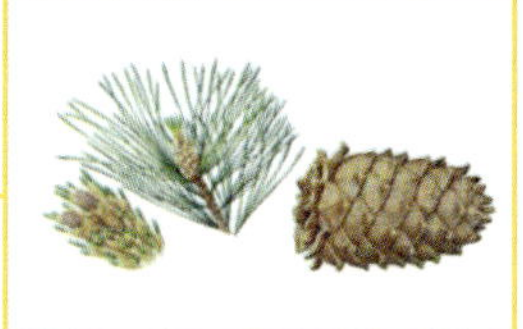

Character:
CONFIDENT, FIRMLY ROOTED; SPIRITUAL STRENGTH

Cedarwood (ALSO CALLED Libanol) is distilled from the wood of the Cedar tree. It is one of the oldest essential oils, used in North Africa as a perfume and medicine. In Ancient Egypt it was used both for preserving mummies and as a massage oil. In the 19th Century it was found to have antiseptic properties.

Aroma: Harmonious, woody, soft.

Properties: Antiseptic; astringent; diuretic; emollient; fungicidal; harmonising; insecticidal; sedative; tonic.

Physical Conditions:
Eliminatory system: cystitis, relieves burning pain; kidney tonic
Respiratory system: helpful with asthma, bronchitis, catarrh, coughs
Musculoskeletal system: may ease chronic arthritic and rheumatic pains
Nervous system: relaxing and calming
Skin: good for acne, oily skin, irritation
Scalp and hair: dandruff, seborrhoea

Mental/Emotional Conditions: Focuses attention when lacking concentration; for scattered thoughts, day-dreaming, living in the future. Calms anxiety and nervous tension.

Other Uses: Combine with Sandalwood for room fragrance for meditation.

Applications: Bath; inhalation; massage; room fragrance.

Blends well with: Sandalwood.

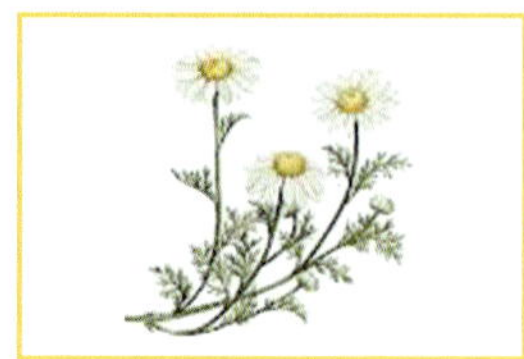

CHAMOMILE *Anthemis Nobilis*

Character:
SOOTHING YET STRONG

Chamomile oil is distilled from the white flower heads of the Chamomile herb. There are many types of Chamomile, including Roman, German and Wild or Moroccan Chamomile. Some are anti-inflammatory, containing azulenes or bisabolene. Wild or Moroccan Chamomile has long been used in the medicine of North Africa.

Aroma: Fresh, herbaceous, tea-like, ardent.

Properties: Antispasmodic; calming; cicatrisant; comforting; febrifuge; sedative of nervous system; warming.

Physical Conditions:
Digestion: colic, colitis, diarrhoea, gastritis, ulcers
Eliminatory system: bedwetting, cystitis, irritable bowel
Hormonal system: decongestant, good for hot flushes
Musculoskeletal system: used for lower back pain, rheumatism and sprains
Nervous system: helpful for depression, headaches, insomnia, when feeling fragile

Mental/Emotional Conditions: For the highly strung and perhaps over-enthusiastic; impulsiveness in helping others; living on nerves and straining energies to their limits.

Applications: Bath; face oil/lotion; facial steaming; footbath; inhalation; massage; room fragrance.

Blends well with: Geranium, Lavender, Ylang Ylang.

CLARY SAGE *Salvia Sclarea*

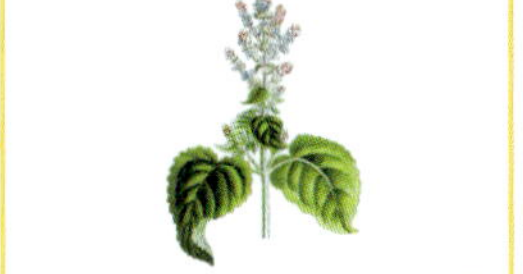

Character:
BENEVOLENT

Clary Sage is distilled from the lilac flowering tops of a biennial herb with large wrinkled leaves, growing in England, Europe, Russia and the USA. It is related to, but different from, the common sage used in cooking. The name *Salvia* derives from the Latin for 'good health' and the word 'clary' meaning 'clear'; the seeds were once used in a remedy to clear particles from the eyes. Clary Sage can have euphoric effects, and from the 16th Century was added to beer by some brewers.

Aroma: Light, spicy, like drying hay.

Properties: Antidepressant; antiseptic; carminative; deodorant; sedative; tonic. Regulatory and balancing. Strongly sedative, but sometimes with euphoric effects.

Physical Conditions:
Hair: encourages growth
Hormonal system: regulates hormones, helpful for pre-menstrual tension and painful periods, also frigidity. Encourages labour*
Musculoskeletal system: relieves cramp, muscle spasm
Nervous system: exhaustion, insomnia from over-work, headaches, migraines
Respiratory system: asthma, throat infections
Skin: excessive perspiration
*Use with caution: can cause excessive bleeding

Mental/Emotional Conditions: Particularly indicated for times of change, domestic, occupational and biological, and when having difficulty in adjusting to changes in life.

Other Uses: Aphrodisiac. Restorative when convalescing.

Applications: Bath; hair oil/rinse; massage; room fragrance.
- Can cause drowsiness; best not used before driving or drinking alcohol.

Blends well with: Rosemary, Ylang Ylang.

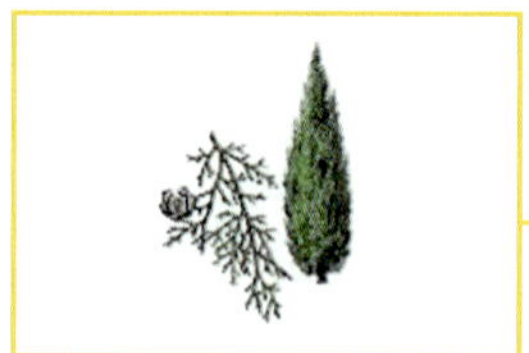

CYPRESS *Cupressus Sempervirens*

Character:
SOLEMN, FIRM, UPRIGHT, ASTRINGENT

Cypress oil is distilled from the wood of the majestic Cypress tree, which grows in Europe, particularly around the Mediterranean. The tree has been venerated since ancient times, and gave its name to the Greek island of Cyprus. It has also been associated with burial grounds since Greek and Roman days, and is traditionally believed to have supplied the wood for Christ's Cross. Known for its astringent properties, the oils is often used today in perfumery, especially men's cosmetics.

Aroma: Refreshing, woody, spicy.

Properties: Antiseptic; antispasmodic; astringent; deodorant; toning; vasoconstrictor.

Physical Conditions:
Circulation: haemorrhoids, nosebleeds, varicose veins, cellulitis
Eliminatory system: bedwetting, frequent urination, excessive perspiration
Hormonal system: hormone imbalance, pre-menstrual tension, heavy periods, painful periods, menopause
Hair and scalp: dandruff with oily scalp
Musculoskeletal system: cramps, rheumatism
Nervous system: warms coldness in nervous system
Respiratory system: asthma, coughs (bronchitis and dry), influenza
Skin: can benefit mature, oily and sweaty skin. Helps heal wounds

Mental/Emotional Conditions: For fear of what others think; inability to withstand pressure from others of more dominant personality.

Other Uses: Insecticide; deodorant; male toiletry.

Applications: Bath; face lotion; facial steaming; hair oil/rinse; inhalation; room fragrance.

Blends well with: Frankincense, Red Grapefruit, Juniper, Lemon.

EUCALYPTUS *Eucalyptus Globulus*

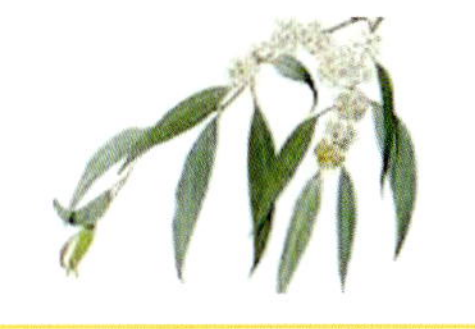

Character:
HARMONISING, VIGOROUS, DEEPLY GROUNDED

Eucalyptus, or Blue Gum is one of the most widely used essential oils; a constituent of cold remedies and inhalants, and strongly antiseptic. The oil is distilled from the blue-green leaves of the Eucalyptus tree, which grows to a great height in warm regions. A native of Tasmania, its leaves were used by the Aboriginals as a dressing for wounds. It was introduced to Europe in the 18th Century.

Aroma: Resinous, camphorous, clear, powerful.

Properties: Analgesic; anti-rheumatic; antiseptic; decongestant; deodorising; energy balancing; insecticidal.

Physical Conditions:
Eliminatory system: cystitis, diarrhoea
Musculoskeletal system: muscular aches and pains, rheumatism (combined with Lemon and Juniper), sciatica
Nervous system: neuralgia
Respiratory system: asthma, bronchitis, catarrh, colds, cold with headache, sinusitis
Skin: burns, inflammatory conditions, insect bites, skin eruptions

Mental/Emotional Conditions: Cools heated emotions; balances extreme moods/highs and lows occurring for no apparent reason; aids concentration.

Other Uses: Insect repellent.

Applications: Bath; inhalation; massage.

Blends well with: Cedarwood, Ginger, Marjoram, Rosemary.

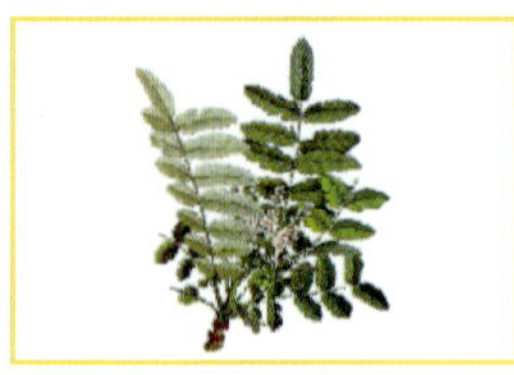

FRANKINCENSE *Boswellia Carterii*

Character:
INSPIRING AND CONTEMPLATIVE, HARMONISING

Frankincense, or Olibanum is distilled from the resin of a small desert tree growing in the Middle East and North Africa. Famous as a birth gift to the infant Jesus, it has had religious and therapeutic uses for centuries. The Ancient Egyptians burned it in religious ceremonies, and also used it in massage and to rejuvenate the skin. Today it is used as an incense in many religions.

Aroma: Spicy, resinous, balsamic, almost lemony.

Properties: Antiseptic; calming; cooling; drying; fortifying; revitalising; stimulating; tonic; uplifting.

Physical Conditions:
Circulation: haemorrhoids, nosebleeds
Digestive system: indigestion
Eliminatory system: cystitis
Nervous system: chilliness
Respiratory system: asthma, bronchitis, catarrh, congested lungs, shortness of breath
Skin: acne scarring, ageing, cracked, oily, wrinkles

Mental/Emotional Conditions: For over-attachment to the past; burn-out, with no conditions; reserves; depression; exhaustion and mental fatigue; fears; insecurity; nightmares; panic.

Other Uses: Aid to medication and spiritual development.

Applications: Bath; face oil/lotion; facial steaming; inhalation; massage; room fragrance.

Blends well with: Cypress, Ginger, Orange, Sandalwood, Tangerine.

GERANIUM *Pelargonium Graveolens*

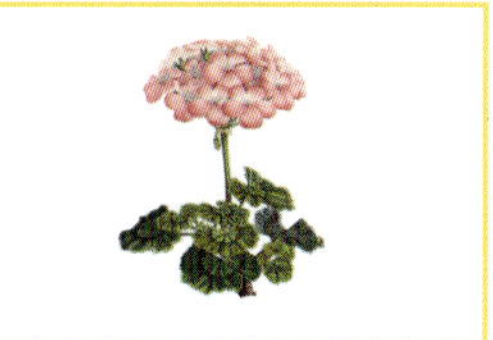

Character:
ADAPTABLE, STRONG WHEN PURE,
SWEETENS WITH DILUTION

Geranium, or Rose Geranium is distilled from the fragrant leaves of the Pelargonium, a herbaceous plant with pink flowers. The oil is often obtained from France, Madagascar, Morocco and other warm climates. Geranium was once used as a general healing herb for wounds, fractures, cholera etc. The oil has beneficial effects on most skin conditions and stimulates the lymphatic system. It is widely used in soaps and perfumes. It is one of the balancing oils; harmonising extreme conditions, both physical and emotional.

Aroma: Sweet, fruity, rose-like.

Properties: Analgesic; antidepressant; astringent; balancing; diuretic; harmonising; insecticidal; tonic; vasoconstrictor.

Physical Conditions:
Circulatory system: a tonic, helps relieve fluid tension and lymphatic congestion
Eliminatory system: a tonic for the liver and kidneys
Hormonal system: regulatory, useful for pre-menstrual tension, painful breasts, irregular or heavy periods, menopausal symptoms
Hair and scalp: balances sebum, helps clear head lice
Nervous system: eases neuralgia and fatigue
*Skin: good for all types of skin conditions including dermatitis, blotches and eczema, and in skin lotion. Effective in mouth and throat infections
*N.B. May irritate some skins; patch-test first

Mental/Emotional Conditions: Antidepressant; quells acute fright, when totally rigid with fear or escalating anxiety when an emergency arises; balances extreme moods.

Applications: Bath; face oil/lotion; facial steaming; hair oil/rinse; inhalation; massage; mouthwash; room fragrance.

Blends well with: Most oils, particularly Cedarwood, Cypress, Red Grapefruit, Lavender, Patchouli, Rosemary.

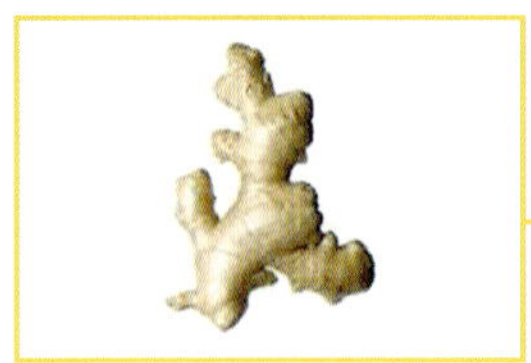

GINGER *Zingiber Officinale*

Character:
WARM, SHARP, PLEASING, CONFIDENT

Ginger comes from Indonesia and sometimes the West Indies. Ginger is mentioned way back in history, not only in Roman times but also in its ancient home in China. Ginger is well known as a spice or condiment and perhaps its original use was as a food preservative and many people know it as a digestive aid. The Ginger herb grows up to 4 feet high or 120cm, but it is the rhizome which gives the spice an essential oil. The Chinese God of Long Life wore a yellow-ginger coloured robe, paying tribute to the use that they saw for the herb. Ginger was introduced into the West Indies by the Spanish to try to steal the trade from the Far East. In fact, very good Ginger oil can be obtained from islands such as Jamaica.

Aroma: Spicy, sharp, warm. Lively and loved.

Properties: Analgesic; antispasmodic; carminative; expectorant; febrifuge; rubefacient; stimulant; stomachic; sudorific.

Physical Conditions:
Digestion: nausea, vomiting, travel sickness, respiratory system. Beneficial for coughs, colds, bronchitis and catarrhal lung conditions
Hormonal system: promotes menstruation and eases menstrual cramps
Loss of appetite: flatulence, constipation
Musculoskeletal system: beneficial in formulations for arthritis, aching muscles and rheumatism
Nervous system: can be useful for those suffering from stomach migraine

Mental/Emotional Conditions: The essential oil has a fiery character that is very useful for those who need their initiative stimulated or their willpower provoked. It aids in all situations where strength, confidence and determination is required. If procrastination is a problem then Ginger will prove very useful. Those who lack confidence or those who have self-doubts that restrain them from actions would do well to use Ginger.

Applications: Massage; inhalation.
- N.B. use with caution - do not use undiluted on the skin as it can cause sensitivity.

Blends well with: Eucalyptus, Frankincense, Lemon, Orange, Patchouli, Sandalwood.

GRAPEFRUIT, Red *Citrus Paridisi*

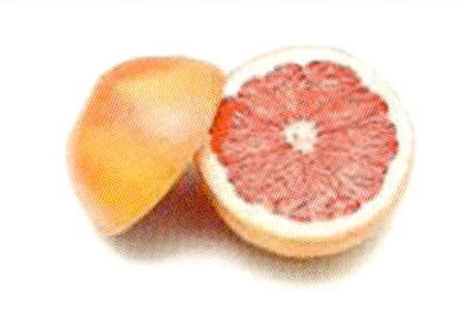

Character:
LIGHTNESS AND PURITY

The Grapefruit what we know from breakfast times has some obscure origins. It is thought to be a hybrid starting with Sweet Orange. It probably started life in the United States, Israel, Cyprus and South Africa. The tree has lovely glossy green leaves and apart from the large yellow fruits has fragrant flowers. In common with other citrus fruits, the essential oil is obtained from the peel of the fruit. Apart from the Grapefruit that we know there are also pink Grapefruits and some essential oils tinged that colour. Many years ago, Grapefruit was known as Shaddock fruit, named after the sea captain who introduced the fruit to the West Indies, and from there to the United States. Grapefruit essential oil is most commonly used in perfumery and soaps as well of course as being a food flavouring agent.

Aroma: Fresh, sweet, citrusy.

Properties: Antidepressant; antiseptic; depurative; diuretic; disinfectant; digestive stimulant; lymphatic decongestant.

Physical Conditions:
Eliminatory system: lymphatic stimulant with detoxifying and diuretic properties. Cellulitis
Musculoskeletal system: rheumatic pain where swelling is present
Skin: stretch marks
Digestion: sluggish appetite, flatulence, abdominal distension, nausea
Circulation: blood purifier
Nervous system: to relieve feelings of tension, frustration, irritability and moodiness

Mental/Emotional Conditions: Red Grapefruit is uplifting and reviving and can be used in states of nervous exhaustion and stress particularly when expectations of others are not fulfilled. Red Grapefruit is the ideal oil for those who comfort eat and for short temper and anger.

Applications: Face oil; facial steaming; massage; room fragrance.

Blends well with: Cypress, Geranium, Juniper, Lemon.

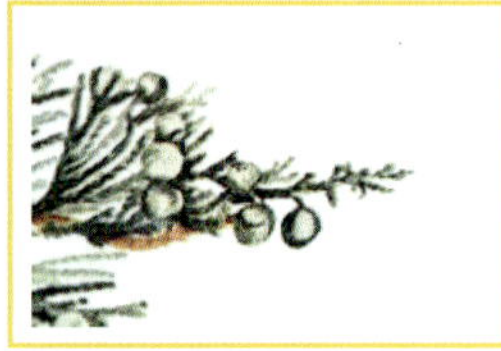

JUNIPER *Juniperus Communis*

Character:
ROUGH, BITTER BUT CONSOLING, STRENGTHENING

Juniper is distilled from the berries or twigs of the Juniper tree, a grey-green leafed tree which grows in many parts of the world, thriving in Arctic conditions. Juniper oil has traditionally been used as an antiseptic by many cultures, and in the past was a constituent of herbal medicines for the plague, cholera, typhoid fever and even diabetes. It has also been noted for its reviving qualities, and today is well known as an ingredient of gin.

Aroma: Green, herbaceous, refreshing.

Properties: Antiseptic; anti-rheumatic; antispasmodic; astringent; cleansing; detoxifying; diuretic; insecticidal; stimulant; tonic.

Physical Conditions:
Circulation: a blood purifier
Digestive system: generally beneficial, detoxifying, cleanses liver after rich food and too much alcohol
**Eliminatory system:* decongestant and diuretic, good for cystitis, painful urination, kidney problems, cellulitis and fluid retention
Musculoskeletal system: good for arthritis, cramps, rheumatism, sciatica
**N.B. Prolonged use may over stimulate the kidneys. Avoid in cases of serious kidney disease

Mental/Emotional Conditions: Helps to lift guilt, despondency, lack of self-worth; for feeling undeserving of love and dissatisfied with physical form. Strengthens and supports: food for people in the caring professions.

Other uses: Hangover; hayfever.

Applications: Bath; footbath; massage; room fragrance.

Blends well with: Frankincense, Red Grapefruit, Rosemary.

KUNZEA *Kunzea Ambigua*

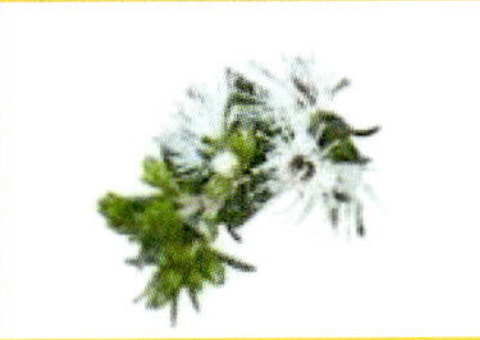

Character:
STRONG AND VIGOROUS, YET KIND

Kunzea is a shrub from Tasmania and southeast Australia that bears sweetly fragrant white flowers. A very healing essential oil with a typically medicinal note that becomes more gentle and spice like as it evaporates. The local name is 'Tick Bush' as it repels insects and grazing animals often seek its shelter. In Australia it has a medical registration for the relief of pain from arthritis and other aches and pains. Useful as a relief for sinusitis and useful against influenza. Mouth and teeth conditions can be treated.

Aroma: Fresh, clean, medicinal, sweetly spice like.

Properties: Analgesic; anti-rheumatic; anti-viral; disinfecting; fungicidal; refreshing.

Physical Conditions:
Musculoskeletal system: rheumatism, aches and pains
Skin: effective against bruising and chilblains, anti-inflammatory,eczema, shingles
Mouth: can be used for ulcers external and internal and gum disease and toothache
Respiratory system: use against sinusitis, bronchitis, common colds

Mental/Emotional Conditions: Relieves anxiety and panic attacks as well as stress and nervous headaches; deep emotional pain is dissipated.

Other uses: Promotes quick repair of soft tissue damage as in sports injury.

Applications: Neat; inhalation; massage; steaming; friction; space fragrance.

Blends well with: Eucalyptus, Cedarwood, Lemon, Cypress.

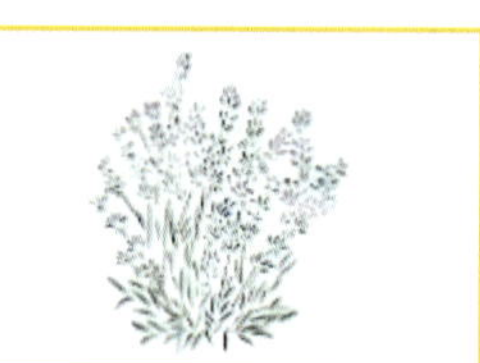

LAVENDER *Lavandula angustifolia, hybrid*

Lavender oils are distilled from the blue flowering spikes of the Lavender bush, just before opening. The plant is widely cultivated in Europe and a hybrid called Lavendin grows wild in the Mediterranean area. The Lavender plant has been used in medicine since ancient times, and was introduced to England by the Romans. It has long been known as an antiseptic and an insecticide, and was known for its skin healing properties. Lavender oil is invaluable in a home first aid kit, particularly for insect stings, cuts and burns. It is the first choice for insomnia and anxiety, and also boosts the immune system. It is also, of course, a popular constituent of perfumes and cosmetic products.

Aroma: Clean, balsamic, light, herbaceous.

Properties: Analgesic; antidepressant; antiseptic; anti-viral; carminative; deodorant; detoxifying; fungicidal; insecticidal; restorative; sedative. Healing for mind and body.

Physical Conditions:
Circulation: relieves chilblains
Eliminatory system: for pain when urinating
Hormonal system: helpful for hot flushes
Hair and scalp: kills headlice; helpful against hair loss
Immune system: stimulates when below par (indicated by chronic or recurrent infections)
Musculoskeletal system: relieves arthritis pain, painful joints and sprains
Nervous system: relaxing and sedative. Excellent for insomnia, tension headaches and migraine, exhaustion
Respiratory system: relieves sore or dry throat
Skin: healing and antiseptic for abscesses, acne, dermatitis, eczema, burns, sunburn, cuts, insect stings and bites

Mental/Emotional Conditions: Excellent for all forms of anxiety and tension. For apprehensiveness with vague fears; nightmares and feelings of panic with inner trembling; fear of the dark.

Other uses: Helpful with tinnitus when sensitive to noise. Counteracts travel sickness.

Applications: Bath; face oil/lotion; facial steaming; footbath; hair oil/rinse; inhalation; massage; room fragrance; a drop or two can be dabbed direct on insect stings; use dilute on burns.

Blends well with: Clary Sage, Eucalyptus, Geranium, Juniper, Patchouli.

LEMON *Citrus Limonum*

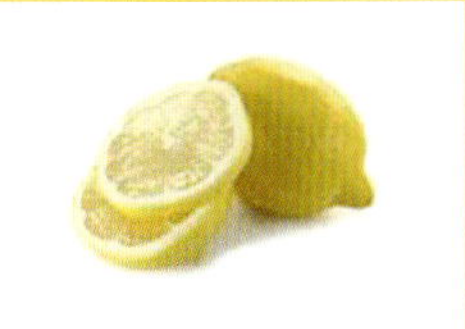

Character:
FRESH, STRONG, VERSATILE. ADDS CHARACTER;
HARMONISES WELL

Lemon oil is pressed from the lemon rind. Several varieties of Lemon tree are grown in warm climates; originating in India it was first brought to Europe by the crusaders, and is widely cultivated in Italy. It has long been used as an antiseptic, particularly for bites by disease-carrying insects. Today it is used as a flavouring in foods and drinks.

Aroma: Fresh, clean, refreshing, lively.

Properties: Anti-infectious; anti-rheumatic; antiseptic; astringent; carminative; detoxifying; diuretic; insecticidal; laxative; stimulating; styptic; tonic; refreshing; uplifting. Acts on the physical, mental and spiritual defence systems.

Physical Conditions:
Circulation: a good tonic, helps to lower high blood pressure, stems nosebleeds and external bleeding
Digestion: improves digestion, balances acidity
Eliminatory system: helpful for cellulitis and fluid retention, generally cleansing and detoxifying
Hair and scalp: cleanses greasy hair
Immune system: stimulates when below par (indicated by chronic or recurrent infections)
Musculoskeletal system: helps relieve aches and pains
Nervous system: soothes neuralgia
Respiratory system: relieves colds, sore throats, influenza and coughs
Skin: clears corns, warts and verrucas, broken veins, clears skin of dead cells

Mental/Emotional Conditions: Refreshing and clarifying; good for feelings of resentment or bitterness about life's experiences; touchiness; when grudging of others' lack of success.

Applications: Bath; face oil/lotion; facial steaming; footbath; hair oil/rinse; inhalation; massage; room fragrance; apply directs to corns, warts and verrucas.
N.B. Dilute well as high dosage may irritate skin or cause photosensitivity.

Blends well with: Chamomile, Eucalyptus, Frankincense, Ginger, Red Grapefruit, Juniper, Lavender, Sandalwood, Ylang Ylang.

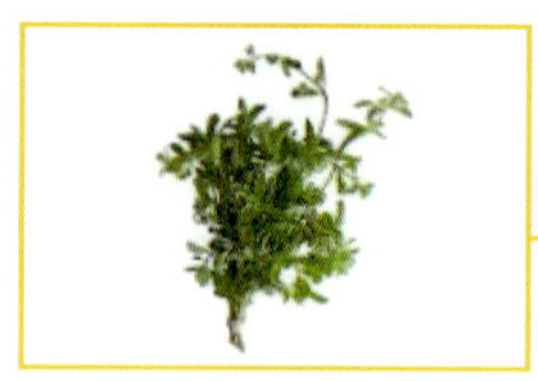

MARJORAM *Origanum Marjorana*

Character:
GENTLE, COMFORTING, WARMING

Marjoram is distilled from the small white flowers of the herb which grows in southern Europe and is widely used in flavouring food. The oil is physically and mentally calming and pain-relieving, useful in rheumatic and back pains, and in promoting the circulation.

Aroma: Warm, herbaceous, with Eucalyptus notes.

Properties: Analgesic; antiseptic; anti-spasmodic; calming; carminative; digestive; laxative; restorative; sedative; tonic.

Physical Conditions:
Digestion: soothing, may help with indigestion, flatulence and constipation
Eliminatory system: a decongestant
Musculoskeletal system: a muscle relaxant, relieves aches and pains, especially when cold and stiff; for stiffness after sport
Nervous system: headaches, migraines, insomnia
Respiratory system: good for bronchitis, chest infections, cold, sinusitis, clears head congestion

Mental/Emotional Conditions: Soothing and relaxing, good when feeling hostile or withdrawn. For those who find it hard to display emotions. Also for mental strain, hyperactivity, irrational thoughts.

Applications: Bath; facial steaming; footbath; inhalation; massage; room fragrance.

Blends well with: Lavender, Lemon.

NEROLINA *Melaleuca Quinquinervia*

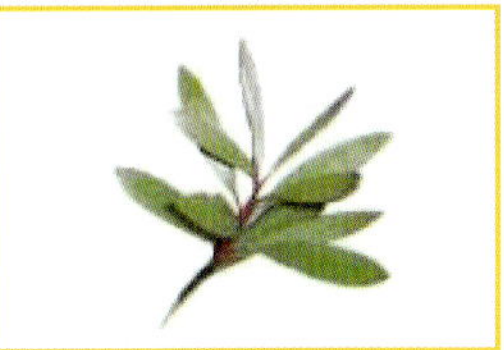

Character:
PLEASING, HAPPY AND PEACEFUL

Nerolina is a common name given to a particular type of essential oil derived from the broad-leaf Paperbark tree found in the swamp and wetlands of the Australian east coast. The main molecules extracted by steam distillation and found in this chemo type are nerolidol and linalool which distinguishes it from other chemotypes of Paperbark such as the cineole rich Niaouli. Melaleucas are commonly called tea trees and Nerolina certainly smells the sweetest resembling Lavender in some ways with similar uses. It is popular in skin care products and as a fixative in aromatherapy blends.

Aroma: Lavender and lilac notes with a clean woody taint.

Properties: Analgesic; antidepressant; anti-viral; restorative; sedative. Healing for mind and body.

Physical conditions:
Hormonal system: useful in menopausal symptoms
Nervous system: useful against insomnia, tension headaches, relaxing and sedative; migraine, exhaustion
Respiratory system: bronchitis, colds, coughs
Skin: acne, dermatitis, burns and sunburn, bites and stings, clears dull skin, detoxifying
Mental/Emotional conditions: Good for all stress and tension situations. Inner trembling with sickness and dizziness, panic attacks, apprehension

Other uses: With a slight wax texture useful as fixative in blends and perfumes and for skin care products.

Applications: Bath; inhalation; steaming; massage; room fragrance; neat on bites but dilute otherwise.

Blends well with: Lavender, Clary Sage, Geranium, Sweet Marjoram, Clove, Nutmeg.

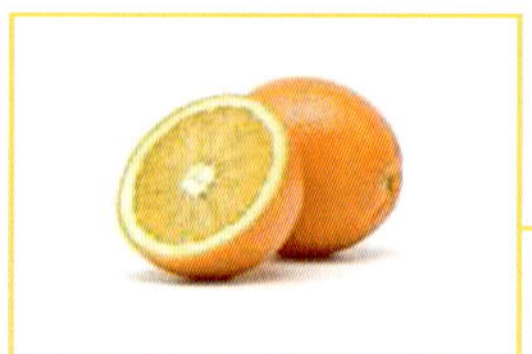

ORANGE *Citrus Sinensis*

Character:
MELLOW, WARMING, SOOTHING, CHEERING

Orange oil is expressed from the zest of the orange fruit; the tree originated in China and today is grown widely in hot climates. It was probably brought to Europe by the Crusaders; later it was taken to California by the early missionaries. The oil is used in perfume and for food flavouring. It works well on the emotions, lifting gloom and depression and encouraging a hopeful outlook.

Aroma: Mellow, fruity, sweet.

Properties: Anticoagulant; antidepressant; antiseptic; antispasmodic; carminative; detoxifying; digestive; sedative; tonic.

Physical Conditions:
Digestion: calms nervous stomach, dyspepsia, gastric spasm, also helpful for both constipation and diarrhoea
Eliminatory system: helps sweat out toxins from skin
Musculoskeletal system: stimulates body tissue repair, relieves muscular aches and pains
Nervous system: a balancing oil, calming and relaxing as needed, can help insomnia
Respiratory system: good for bronchitis, colds
Skin: good for ageing, dry skin, and dermatitis

Mental/Emotional Conditions: Very good for depression, hopelessness, sadness and lack of joy; energises when apathetic, resigned and unable to make necessary changes. Good during periods of hard work.

Other uses: Aids absorption of Vitamin C; brings down temperature; energises.

Applications: Bath; face oil/lotion; inhalation; massage; room fragrance.
*N.B. dilute well as high dosage may irritate skin or cause photosensitivity.

Blends well with: Ginger, Rosemary, Ylang Ylang.

PATCHOULI *Pogostemon Cablin*

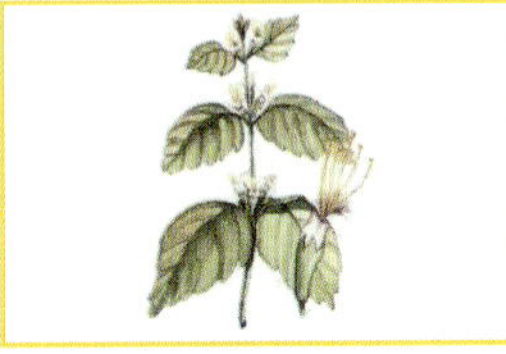

Character:
STRENGTH, EARTHINESS, RICH

Patchouli will be remembered by all those who love the '60s and '70s. Patchouli was common among all the Hippie generation. It was also popular in Victorian England because fabrics and shawls imported from India were scented with Patchouli as a form of moth proofing but the buyers just loved the aroma. Today Patchouli mainly comes from Indonesia. It is actually a small herb and the essential oil is distilled from the dried leaves. The herb can be harvested up to three times a year but the best oil comes from leaves which are actually harvested in the rainy season. Patchouli is also very popular in the perfumers' repertoire. It underpins many oriental type perfumes and is valued not only for its earthy and exotic fragrance but also because it acts as a fixative in perfume materials. This use speaks of its tenacity and strength. The aroma of Patchouli is said to improve with age and Patchouli at its best has a distinctive dry note, or feel, to it.

Aroma: Sweet, warm, earthy with a hint of spice. Drier with age.

Properties: Antidepressant; antiseptic; aphrodisiac; deodorant; sedative; cicatrisant.

Physical Conditions:
Eliminatory system: useful for fluid retention and where diuretic properties are required; cellulite, deodorising
Skin: as a tissue regenerator - especially good for cracked, rough or sore skin, useful against acne, eczema and similar skin conditions
Hair: a general tonic for scalp disorders
Circulation: in combination with other oils such as citrus it is useful as a vascular decongestant and suitable for varicose veins

Mental/Emotional Conditions: Patchouli is said to be grounding and integrating. It is useful for anyone who feels outside of reality. It can be helpful to anyone who feels overactive and has quietening and relaxing effects. Similarly it can be helpful for those suffering from sexual anxiety, frigidity or impotence. For those shattered by work it can be a rest and relaxation bringing people back to being in touch with themselves.

Other uses: Patchouli has been used as a meditation aid and for providing inspiration.

Applications: Face oil/lotion; facial steaming; massage; room fragrance; bathing.

Blends well with: Geranium, Ginger, Lavender, Rosewood, Sandalwood, Ylang Ylang.

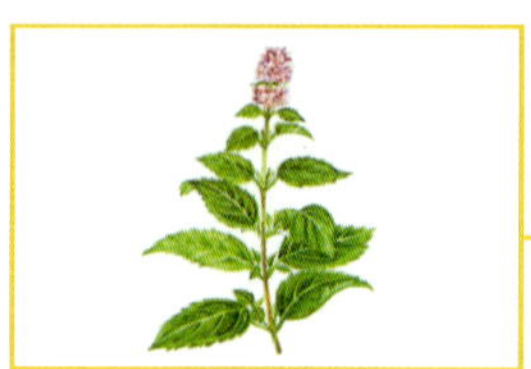

PEPPERMINT *Mentha Piperita*

Character:
HOT AND COLD; STIMULATING.

Peppermint is distilled from the whole herb, an invasive herbaceous plant. There are many species, including Mint and Spearmint, all of which are used widely in medicines and in flavouring confectionery, toothpaste, etc. In Greek mythology, Mentha was a nymph who was pursued by Pluto, the God of the underworld. His jealous wife trod her into the ground, but Pluto ensured her survival by transforming her into the herb. Peppermint has been used for centuries for digestive problems; in warm climates peppermint tea is commonly drunk after meals. The oil is also good for aches and pains, and respiratory congestion. It is rich in menthol, often used in embrocations and inhalants. While best known for digestive and respiratory conditions, it has other lesser known but very useful applications.

Aroma: Minty, fresh, slightly sweet, powerful.

Properties: Anti-inflammatory; analgesic; antiseptic; antispasmodic; astringent; carminative; clarifying; cooling; detoxifying; deodorising; pain-relieving; refreshing; stimulating; vasoconstrictor.

Physical Conditions:
Digestion: useful for bad breath, colic, constipation, diarrhoea, flatulence, food poisoning, gastritis, indigestion, nausea, nervous dyspepsia, vomiting
Eliminatory system: irritable bowel, encourages perspiration
Musculoskeletal system: anti-inflammatory for muscle aches and pains, excellent for aching feet
Nervous system: pain relieving, eases headaches, migraines
Respiratory system: clearing for colds, flu and sinus congestion, laryngitis
Skin: cooling for inflammation, sunburn, irritation, can help dermatitis and ringworm. Balances greasy skin, helps remove blackheads

Mental/Emotional Conditions: For shyness and hypersensitivity to many things; for those dominated by strong likes and dislikes.

Other uses: Travel sickness, shock, faintness, vertigo.

Applications: Bath; face oil/lotion; facial steaming; footbath; hair oil/rinse; inhalation; massage; mouthwash; room fragrance.
N.B. Use with caution and dilute well, as this oil is extremely powerful and could cause irritation of skin and mucus membranes.

Blends well with: Best left alone as it overwhelms other essences.

ROSEMARY *Rosmarinus Officinalis*

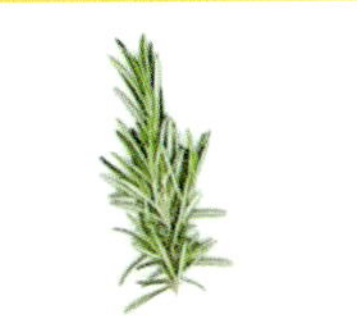

Character:
VIGOROUS PENETRATING, STIMULATING.

Rosemary is distilled from the needle-like leaves of the Evergreen bush. It is also a popular kitchen herb. Originating in Asia, Rosemary now grows in Europe, particularly the south, and is cultivated for oil in France and Tunisia. Rosemary was sacred to the Ancient Greeks and Romans who used it in incense and as a symbol of regeneration; in 14th Century Europe it was believed to have rejuvenating powers and was an ingredient of Hungary Water, a very popular toilet water. Rosemary oil is known as a blood and lymph stimulant, as it stimulates the local blood supply and is excellent for aches and pains. It has also long been valued as a brain stimulant; the ancient Romans wore Rosemary sprigs behind the ear to aid concentration and memory. It has also been used with some success to treat baldness and falling hair; while it may not affect all cases, it is certainly worth trying.

Aroma: Strong, woody, camphoraceous, refreshing.

Properties: Analgesic; antidepressant; anti-rheumatic; antiseptic; antispasmodic; tonic; astringent; carminative; cleansing; clearing; digestive; diuretic; invigorating; stimulating.

Physical Conditions:
Circulation: boosts circulation, heart tonic and stimulant, normalises low blood pressure. Relieves chilblains and chilliness
Digestion: stimulates digestive process
Eliminatory system: boosts liver and kidney function, good for constipation, cystitis and hangovers
Hormonal system: may relieve menstrual pain and fluid retention
Hair and scalp: excellent tonic may be helpful for baldness and falling hair, good for dandruff and oil scalp
Musculoskeletal system: very useful for aches, pains, sprains, muscle fatigue and rheumatism
Nervous system: clears headaches, mental fatigue, migraine, stimulates brain & memory
Skin: good for oily skin, boosts circulation

Mental/Emotional Conditions: Clearing and stimulating for feelings of disorientation, indecision and lethargy; feelings of inadequacy; feeling overwhelmed by responsibilities.

Applications: Bath; face oil/lotion; facial steaming; footbath; hair oil/rinse; inhalation; massage; room fragrance. *N.B. Use with caution if suffering from high blood pressure, hypertension and/or insomnia, or epilepsy.

Blends well with: Cedarwood, Frankincense, Geranium, Juniper, Orange, Tangerine.

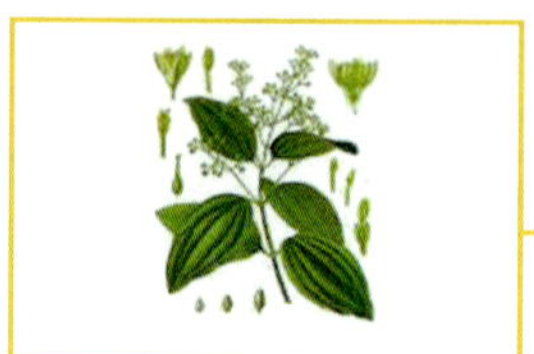

ROSEWOOD *Aniba Parviflora*

Character:
SOFT SWEETNESS WITH BODY, BALANCING

Rosewood, or Bois de Rose is distilled from the wood of a South American tree. Its main uses are psychological; it has a balancing effect, uplifting when lethargic and overburdened, soothing anxiety, irritability and inner tension. It is believed to be beneficial to mature skin as a cell stimulant and tissue regenerator and can be helpful with problems of ageing.

Aroma: Floral with spicy undertones.

Properties: Antiseptic; antidepressant; aphrodisiac; balancing; calming; deodorant grounding; regenerative; stabilising; stimulating; uplifting.

Physical Conditions:
Digestion: nausea with anxiety
Eliminatory system: deodorant
Hormonal system: may be helpful for loss of libido, frigidity, impotence
Immune system: boosts body's defence system, helpful for chronic complaints
Nervous system: balancing and stabilising, neurotic, sedative, may relieve headaches accompanied by nausea
Respiratory system: good for throat infections
Skin: cell and tissue stimulant, rejuvenating for dry skin and ageing skin pigmentation. Relieves insect bites

Mental/Emotional Conditions: Good for rigid attitudes; when over-critical of others, lacking empathy, unyielding to others or to circumstances; for inner tension and rigidity.

Other uses: Aphrodisiac; insect repellent.

Applications: Face oil/lotion; footbath; massage; room fragrance.

Blends well with: Cedarwood, Frankincense, Geranium, Patchouli, Rosemary, Tangerine, Ylang Ylang.

SANDALWOOD *Santalum Album*

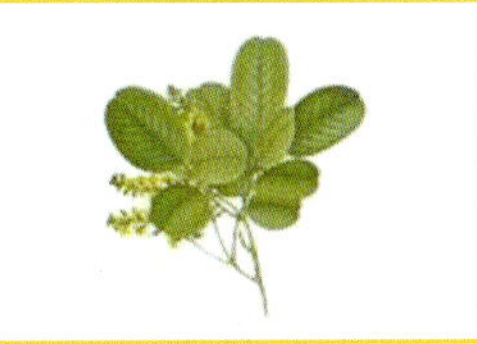

Character:
PERSISTENT, SENSUOUS

Sandalwood, or Bois de Santal is distilled from the heartwood of an Evergreen Indian tree which is parasitic on other trees. Sandalwood has been popular for centuries in furniture and casket making, as well as incense, and was used to build Indian temples. The Ancient Egyptians used Sandalwood oil in embalming and medicines. It is valued as incense today in India, China and Japan. In India it has strong spiritual connotations, being burned at weddings and funerals; it is also used medicinally for genito-urinary problems. Believed to encourage self-expression, Sandalwood is very helpful for laryngitis and sore throats. It is exceptionally long-lasting, and is used as a fixative in perfumes.

Aroma: Warm, rich, sweet, woody.

Properties: Antiseptic; antispasmodic; aphrodisiac; astringent; carminative; diuretic; healing; regenerative; relaxing; soothing; tonic.

Physical Conditions:
Eliminatory system: alleviates cystitis, lymphatic decongestant
Hormonal system: a sensual stimulant, it can be helpful with sexual problems
Immune system: boosts immune deficiency, characterised by persistent infections
Nervous system: very relaxing for nervous tension
Respiratory system: useful for laryngitis, chest, throat and lung infections, bronchitic and dry coughs
Skin: good for ageing, dry skins; relieves itching, inflammation and dry eczema. Antiseptic for acne, boils, cuts and wounds

Mental/Emotional Conditions: Balancing for people who are possessive and manipulative, who like their own way; for difficulty in forgiving; for those who do things for others but fear a lack of return. Helpful with obsessional attitudes, worry about past and future, feeling unsupported. Brings peace and acceptance. May be helpful for sexual anxiety.

Other uses: An aid to meditation, and spiritual development, associated with the 'third eye' and development of intuition.

Applications: Bath; face oil/lotion; facial steaming; inhalation; massage; room fragrance.

Blends well with: Cypress, Frankincense, Ginger, Lavender, Lemon, Patchouli, Ylang Ylang.

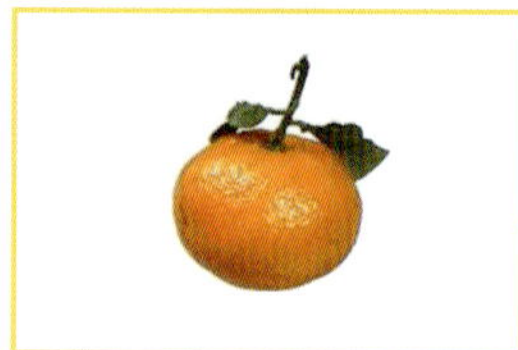

TANGERINE/MANDARIN *Citrus Reticulata*

Character:
REFINED, SOFT, CHEERFUL, UPLIFTING, SWEET

Tangerine or Mandarin oil is expressed from the zest of the citrus fruit, which originated in China and is now cultivated in other warm climates, including the USA and Sicily. Tangerine and Mandarin trees come from the same botanical source. Tangerine oil is a yellow-gold colour, with a light blue fluorescence in the best quality oils (quality depends on the time of harvest). Like many oils, Tangerine can be both relaxing and tonic, according to needs. Its medicinal properties are similar to those of Orange.

Aroma: Sweet, fruity, tangy.

Properties: Antiseptic; antispasmodic; cheering; sedative; soothing; stomachic; tonic; unwinding; uplifting.

Physical Conditions:
Cardiovascular system: calms excitation and cardiovascular erethism which often goes with indigestion
Circulation: tonifies the peripheral circulation in the extremities, revives tired and aching limbs
Digestion: a digestive tonic, good for gastric complaints including constipation, diarrhoea and flatulence, stimulates bile excretion, thereby activating the stomach and liver
Nervous system: sedative, hypnotic, soothes and relaxes, good for insomnia
Skin: a useful skin tonic, encouraging circulation

Mental/Emotional Conditions: Good for dejection, depression, emotional emptiness; regrets for ageing and loss of the past; feeling watered down.

Other uses: Cheering and uplifting; popular as a room fragrance in hospices.

Applications: Bath; face oil/lotion; footbath; massage; room fragrance.

Blends well with: Chamomile, Clary Sage, Geranium, Lavender, Lemon.

TEA TREE *Melaleuca Alternifolia*

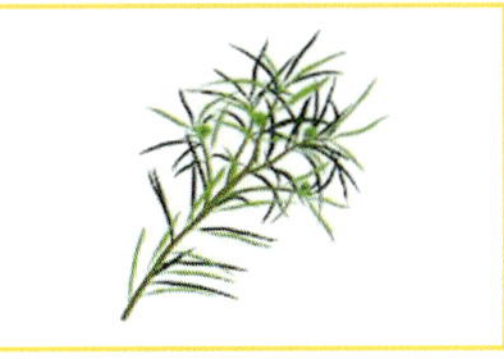

Character:
VIGOROUS, REVITALISING, REGENERATING

Tea Tree oil is distilled from the leaves and branches of the Tea Tree, a small tree belonging to the Myrtle family, and a native of the marshland of New South Wales. It acquired its name when Captain Cook's sailors used it to brew up a substitute for tea. Tea Tree oil is a powerful antiseptic and fungicide and boosts the depleted immune system. Its wide range of medicinal uses have been verified by research. In the 1920s and '30s, laboratory research in Australia confirmed that was not only a very strong antiseptic but non-toxic and non-irritant. A report noted that it dissolved pus, leaving infected wounds clean. During World War II it was issued in army topical first aid kits but the development of antibiotics led to a decline in its use. A 1972 study showed that that Tea Tree oil was effective in many foot problems, including athlete's foot, corns, bunions and other fungal infections. It has also been found helpful with Candida albicans and chronic cystitis. It is an ideal first aid home remedy; for serious chronic conditions, readers should consult a qualified practitioner.

Aroma: Medicinal, penetrating.

Properties: Powerful antiseptic; anti-viral; bactericide; cleansing; detoxifying; fungicidal; insecticidal; purifying; stimulating.

Physical Conditions:
Eliminatory system: used to treat urinary infections, cystitis and Candida
Hair and scalp: impetigo, headlice, dry scalp and dandruff
Immune system: activates the white blood cells to fight infection
Respiratory system: combats infections of the throat, lungs and ears; bad breath
Skin: very cleansing, antiseptic for acne, boils, cuts, wounds, bites; effective with corns, warts, verrucas, fights fungal infections (e.g. Athlete's foot, ringworm), soothes and heals irritating/itchy conditions - chicken pox rash, psoriasis, impetigo, nappy rash, genital itching, pruritus; treatment for mouth ulcers and gum/mouth infections

Mental/Emotional Symptoms: Refreshing and revitalising; for feelings of uncleanliness; for over-preoccupation with detail.

Applications: Bath; face oil/lotion; facial steaming; footbath; hair oil/rinse; inhalation; massage; mouthwash; room fragrance.

Blends well with: Best used alone.

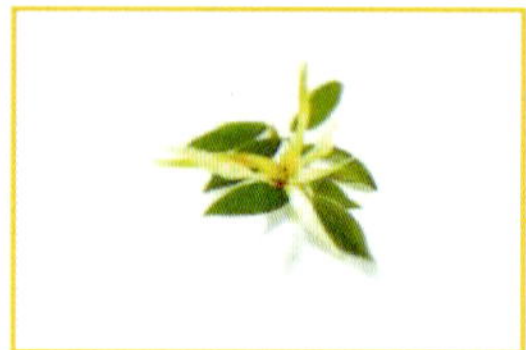

YLANG YLANG *Cananga Odorata*

Character:
VOLUPTUOUS, SENSUAL, EXOTIC, YET REASSURING

Ylang Ylang, 'The Flower of Flowers' is distilled from the yellow flowers of a tree growing in Indonesia, the Philippines and Madagascar. It is also known as the 'Perfume Tree'. In the South Seas women combine the oil with coconut oil to dress their hair, and in Indonesia the blossoms are spread on the beds of honeymoon couples. The oil is used in expensive perfumes. While Ylang Ylang has physical properties, its main effects are on the emotions, and it is known as an aphrodisiac. It is also reassuring and confidence building.

Aroma: Heavy, sweetly narcotic, floral.

Properties: Antidepressant, aphrodisiac, calming, euphoric, sensual, sedative, uplifting.

Physical Conditions:
Circulation: calming for tachycardia, reduces high blood pressure, regulates adrenaline flow
Hormonal system: balances the hormones; a uterine tonic. May help keep breasts firm. Helpful for sexual problems
Hair and scalp: Tonic, promotes hair growth
Nervous system: has relaxing effect
Skin: balances both dry and oily skins

Mental/Emotional Conditions: Calms anger, fear, frustration, irritability; is believed to act on the emotional heart centre, healing feelings of guilt, jealousy, resentment and selfishness. Also helpful in times of change.

Applications: Bath; face oil/lotions; hair oil/rinse; massage; room fragrance.

Blends well with: Clary Sage, Geranium, Lavender, Lemon, Orange, Patchouli.

FURTHER READING

Liquid Sunshine	Jan Kuśmirek - Floramicus, 2002
Fragrant Earth Desk Reference	Jan Kuśmirek - Floramicus, 2003
Aromatherapy: an A-Z	Patricia Davis - C.W. Daniel & Co. Ltd., 1999
Aromatherapy: A Guide for Home Use	Christine Westwood - Amberwood Publishing Ltd., 1991
Aromatherapy for Women	Maggie Tisserand - Thorsons Publishing, 1999
Aromatherapy: Massage with Essential Oils	Christine Wildwood - Element, 1991
The Aromatherapy Workbook	Shirley Price - Thornsons Publishing Group., 1998
The Practice of Aromatherapy	Jean Valnet - C.W. Daniel & Co., 1980
The Art of Aromatherapy	Robert Tisserand - C.W. Daniel & Co. Ltd., 1977
The Book of Massage	Linda Lidell - Ebury Press, 1991
The Complete Book of Massage	Clare Maxwell-Hudson - Dorling-Kindersley, 1988
The Directory of Essential Oils	Wanda Sellar - C.W. Daniel & Co., 1994
The Encyclopaedia of Essential Oils	Julia Lawless - Thorsons Publishing Group, 2002
The Fragrant Pharmacy	Valerie Ann Worwood - Bantam, 1991
Practical Aromatherapy: How to Use Essential Oils to Restore Vitality	Shirley Price - Thorsons Publishing Group, 1994

EDUCATION

Education is paramount. I recommend the following reputable schools:

Fragrant Studies Japan
K's Minami Aoyama Building 1F, Minami Aoyama 6-6-20, Minato-Ku,
Tokyo, 107-0062, Japan

Fragrant Earth Academy
21 Beckery Road, Glastonbury, Somerset, BA6 9NX, UK

WHERE TO FIND AN AROMATHERAPIST

The following organisations will supply lists of qualified Aromatherapists.
Please enclose stamped addressed envelopes with your enquiries.

The International Federation of Aromatherapists
20A The Mall, Ealing Broadway, London, W5 2PJ, UK

**The International Federation of Professional
Aromatherapists**
82 Ashby Road, Hinckley, Leicestershire, LE10 1SN, UK

The Register of Qualified Aromatherapists
P.O. Box 3431, Danbury, Chelmsford, Essex CM3 4UA, UK

The Aromatherapy Organisations Council
P.O. Box 19834, London SE25 6WF, UK

National Association for Holistic Aromatherapy
P.O. Box 1868, Banner Elk, North Carolina, 28604, USA

Aroma Environment Association of Japan
3-2-11-5F Kyobashi, Chuo-ku, Tokyo, 104-0031, Japan

STOCKISTS

The best essential oils come from a very small number of companies and I recommend:

Fragrant Earth International Ltd.
Unit 21 Beckery Road, Glastonbury, Somerset, BA6 9NX
Tel: +44 (0)1458 831216   Fax: +44 (0)1458 831361

Fragrant Earth World Japan Ltd.
K's Minami Aoyama Building 3F, 6-6-20 Minami Aoyama,
Minato-Ku, Tokyo, 102-0062, Japan
Tel: + 81(3) 5766 6056   Fax: +81(3) 5766 6094

Pranarôm International s.a.
Avenue des Artisans, 37-7822 Ghislenghien, Belgium
Tel: +32(0)68 264 364   Fax: +32(0)68 331 895

Primavera Life GmbH
Naturparadies 1, D-87466 Oy-Mittelberg, Germany
Tel: +49(0)8366 8988 0   Fax: +49(0)8366 8988 4099

For an up-to-date list of stockists, please visit my website, www.jankusmirek.com.